MD Aware

Stephen Liben • Tom A. Hutchinson

MD Aware

A Mindful Medical Practice Course Guide

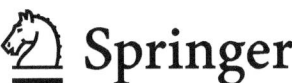 Springer

Stephen Liben
McGill Programs in Whole Person Care
McGill University
Montreal, QC
Canada

Tom A. Hutchinson
McGill Programs in Whole Person Care
McGill University
Montreal, QC
Canada

ISBN 978-3-030-22429-5 ISBN 978-3-030-22430-1 (eBook)
https://doi.org/10.1007/978-3-030-22430-1

This Springer imprint is published by the registered company Springer Nature Switzerland AG
The registered company address is: Gewerbestrasse 11, 6330 Cham, Switzerland

"I'm not a teacher: only a fellow traveler of whom you asked the way. I pointed ahead – ahead of myself as well as you."
— *George Bernard Shaw*

Preface

This book describes the MMP course that emerged as an answer to our years-long conversation on the question, "How can we teach medical students what it has taken each of us decades to learn for ourselves?" We took the best, most impactful learning experiences we ourselves have had and put them together into a course that would be specifically helpful to pre-clerkship medical students. Our intention is to have students experience for themselves the transformational impact of mindful whole person care that we have each seen, time and time again, as a path to healing for both the cared-for and the caregiver.

The experience of teaching this course is like no other that we have ever taught; as one of our colleagues has said, "teaching MMP is both the most rewarding and most difficult teaching I have ever done." We wrote this book because we have been asked repeatedly to "give out the MMP course outline" and we have steadfastly resisted doing so, knowing that to offer the teaching templates alone, without elaborating on how to apply them, would be like teaching someone to cook with only a simple list of ingredients and no other directions in hand.

Each of the chapters that describe the seven MMP classes was written by either one or the other author. Each of us has our own personal style of teaching and writing, and we wanted each to be free to write in our own personal voice. This way, you, the reader, have the opportunity to compare and contrast how the different writing styles resonate with your own personal teaching approach.

As you read, keep in mind that each chapter that describes a class is divided into numbered sections that correspond with the numbers found on the teaching template at the end of each chapter. We have one suggestion as to how to read and use this book: we recommend that once you have read through the book, you then use the end-of-chapter templates, as we ourselves do, as a one-page in-hand guide while teaching each class. Before we teach a class, we read through the relevant chapter and rehearse what we intend to say and do for each learning exercise. While teaching a class, we then use the class template to help keep us on track.

Teaching this course can be challenging (and you will certainly be challenged by students), intense, interesting, and fun. It may be a platitude, but it nonetheless has been true for us that we learn as much if not more than the students we are teaching.

We wish you well on your own teaching and learning journey...

Montreal, QC, Canada   Stephen Liben
                                                                        Tom A. Hutchinson

Acknowledgments

We would like to acknowledge the leadership of McGill University's Faculty of Medicine, the Dean, David Eidelman and the Executive Director Pascale Mongrain for their very generous and consistent support to McGill Programs in Whole Person Care, where our Mindful Medical Practice course was envisioned and developed. We would also like to thank the former Associate Dean Robert Primavesi and the current Associate Dean for Undergraduate Medical Education Beth-Ann Cummings who provided the opening and support necessary for us to launch and continue to teach our course. We thank our colleagues in Whole Person Care, in particular Krista Lawlor and Mark Smilovitch, who played an important role in the development of the course; we would also like to thank Patricia Dobkin, Steven Jordan, and Simon Rousseau, and in addition Joanna Caron and Allen Steverman, who are currently instructors in the course. A special thanks to our students who have been so open to our teaching and a particular acknowledgment of those students who gave their permission to use the transcript of class 6 for chapter 10 and their essays for chapter 12. We are grateful to others who have inspired our mindfulness work with medical students: Saki Santorelli from the University of Massachusetts, Ronald Epstein from the University of Rochester, and Craig Hassed from Monash University. We thank Richard Lansing and Megan Ruzomberka from Springer for facilitating the publication of our work. Finally, a very special thanks to Angelica Todireanu who did all the painstaking detailed work in putting together the manuscript for the book.

Montreal   Tom A. Hutchinson
April 2, 2019   Stephen Liben

Contents

Chapter 1
Introduction

Tom A. Hutchinson and Stephen Liben

MD Aware?

A nurse takes the temperature of a hospitalized 8-year-old boy with a diagnosis of acute lymphoblastic leukemia and finds he has shaking chills and a new fever. The nurse knows this may require starting antibiotics immediately so she/he informs the ward physician and then documents the interaction in the medical chart as "new fever, 39.2 oral, and shaking chills at 19:00, MD aware." The MD has been informed, but is the MD really aware of how ominous this fever might be in this child at this time? Was the MD paying attention when the nurse was letting her/him know of the new finding, or was she/he distracted by another acute emergency or by being too hungry, tired, or overwhelmed? How can we teach the awareness skills of attentional focus, emotional regulation, and curiosity in a busy and often hyperstimulating clinical environment? If it was possible, wouldn't it then be critically important to teach physicians how to be more aware of themselves, the medical contexts they are in, and of the other person – the patient in front of them? We believe it is possible to teach and learn these skills, and the course we have designed to do so is detailed in this book.

Why Read This Book and Who Is It for?

This book has been written for anyone who teaches medicine. While the Mindful Medical Practice (MMP) course as detailed in the book has been designed to teach undergraduate medical students, we have used individual classes taken exactly as they are described in this course to teach both residents in training and physicians who have been in practice for many years. One way the book can be used is to set up an MMP course in a medical school. Everything that is needed to set up such a course is in this book, and our motivation for writing was to respond to requests for

© Springer Nature Switzerland AG 2020
S. Liben, T. A. Hutchinson, *MD Aware*,
https://doi.org/10.1007/978-3-030-22430-1_1

such a detailed course description. But this book is more than a "how to teach MMP" instruction manual. Integrating contemplative practices into medical education is a new way to bring experiential learning to medical students, and we would be remiss if we did not explain why doing so has so much potential.

"The good physician treats the disease; the great physician treats the patient who has the disease." –William Osler.

What people want when they bring a problem to their doctor is "someone who will provide competent medical care and treat him/her seriously as a person" [1, p., 3]. This sounds deceptively simple and yet is most often exactly what patients do not get when they enter the increasingly corporate consumerist profit-based world of hospitals and clinics. Whole person care is what we call the opposite of the reductionist view of medicine that sees doctors only as skilled technicians fixing or replacing body parts of patients seen as broken machines. Whole person care is exactly what those in palliative care found was the missing element that explained why even though none of their patients were cured, many were healed. People are not machines, and well-being and healing are not necessarily related to how well the body is functioning.

Whole person care, as described in the coauthor's (TAH) two books [1, 2], does not leave anything out of the clinical encounter. Whatever the patient brings into the room is open for discussion and evaluation, including all of what is wanted and hoped for, as well as all that is not wanted and feared. The whole person care physician has an awareness of not only their potentially helpful and arduously learned medical knowledge, skills, and attitudes but also of their own human limitations, their ignorance, lack of skill, and unhelpful attitudes. Simply put, to treat the patient as a whole person, the physician needs to bring to awareness their whole personhood. How do we educate physicians to be up to this task, to be ready to engage with anything that might come up in a whole person care-based clinical encounter?

Teaching physicians how to bring their whole personhood into the clinical encounter, to be aware of themselves, the context, and the patient in front of them, requires an education that shows them what this might be like for them, not one that tells them what they should theoretically be doing. The MMP course we describe in this book is one way to show, rather than tell, learning doctors how they themselves can bring a specific type of awareness, a mindful awareness of their whole personhood, to the service of their patients. How can whole person care be taught to physicians? It will not surprise the reader that our response is that to teach whole person care means that teachers need to bring their whole personhood, what they know about themselves, their medical expertise (contexts), and what they have learned about patients, as well as all that they don't know, into the classroom. Teaching MMP is, as our colleagues who have taught with us for the past 5 years have told us, unlike teaching any other course. Teaching MMP requires specific skills (see Chap. 2: Whole Person Teaching and Learning) in addition to a willingness to relearn what was thought to already be known. The MMP teachers are, like whole person care physicians, open to bringing all of who they are into the classroom.

Why Teach MMP? No Other Options?

How do physicians learn to listen to patients, to bring their attention back when they are tired, hungry, bored, restless, or distracted? How do we teach physicians to both know and have strategies to avoid the most common human cognitive errors of anchoring, availability bias, confirmation bias, status quo bias, overconfidence, stereotyping (of self and other), as well as the behavioral effects on decision-making induced by the increased awareness of mortality which is an inevitable accompaniment of medical practice? How do we teach and how do we learn to be empathic and caring (even and especially when we "don't feel like it"), to be with suffering, and to be compassionate? How do we go beyond citing depressing statistics on burnout and substance abuse to students on one PowerPoint slide after another and instead show them how to increase resilience and find meaning in the clinical care of patients? These are not simple concepts that can be learned in the same way that the differential diagnosis for a 2-week-old with fever is internalized and can later be recalled on demand. Unlike learning facts, such as lists of differential diagnoses, learning to be skilled, helpful physicians means experiencing the thoughts, physical sensations, and emotions that arise in the moment as *information* that can then be examined. Is this thought really true? What might this emotion that is arising be telling me and how might it be helpful to both my patient and myself?

This book will describe not only the "how" and "what" of the course but also the "why," as well as some of the unique challenges that teachers may face when using contemplative practices in a nonelective, compulsory, undergraduate course for medical students. Teaching this course is less about the "what" that is being taught, the facts, the kinds of cognitive details that can be tested in multiple-choice exams (although there are indeed specific facts to be learned and tested for in this course), and is more about the "how" teaching and learning develop. In this way, the course is more akin to how teaching and learning occur in the clinical setting, where what is being taught in classic mentor-guided patient encounters is not just "facts" but a multimodal experience that engages all the senses and includes, but is not exclusive to, cognitive facts and therefore is not just learnable by reading books or memorizing facts. A physician walking into a patient's room and meeting another human being in distress (i.e., a patient) requires much more than dealing with cognitive facts (while, at the same time, facts remain important). There are the external smells, sounds, and sights that include nonverbal body communication, as well as the physician's awareness of their own internal thoughts, physical sensations, and emotions that they bring with them from whatever they were experiencing before they entered the room and that then evolve moment to moment. As we will show, developing a nonjudgmental awareness of thoughts, physical sensations, and emotions is important both because it is *information* that the physician can use to help guide diagnostic and therapeutic intuitions and because it is also an essential learnable capacity in avoiding burnout, building resiliency, and finding meaning in clinical work.

Educating the Good Doctor

A good doctor has the knowledge and skills of an applied scientist coupled to the attitudes of a humanist concerned with human flourishing [3]. We make a distinction between learning what is *complicated* versus what is *complex*. *Complicated* concepts are processes that may have many steps but when followed lead to predictable outcomes. The best evidence of the most effective steps to take in a cardiac arrest has been put into a complicated algorithm. What is most required in a cardiac arrest is that the algorithm is followed, and to this end, many physicians carry the algorithm with them on a printed resuscitation card. After a cardiac arrest, the question is whether the algorithm was followed, and the complicated process can be broken down into quantifiable and assessable logical sequential steps. A *complex* process, however, such as how to motivate a patient who is otherwise feeling well to take their antihypertension medication, is not reproducible, is nonlinear, and does not follow a step-by-step logical sequence that can be easily assessed and reproduced. There is no one script that can be told to a patient to ensure medication compliance, and what might be helpful to say to one patient might be the opposite of what is needed for another. One could say that most person-to-person communication is a complex nonlinear, not easily reproducible, and unstable process. For complex clinical problems, what is needed is less the memorization of facts and algorithms and more a method of assessing in the moment and based on best evidence and current understandings, what might be the helpful next step for this patient at this time. Complex problems are the foundation of clinical medicine. The so-called "classic textbook cases" of disease that may be complicated but are predictably not complex are so uncommonly encountered that when a patient presents with a "typical case," there is often a lineup of medical students to see for themselves what a classic case looks like because their everyday experience is seeing patients with everything but the "classic" case presentation.

The good doctor is able to be present to what is happening in a particular way, which we are calling a mindful awareness. Such mindful awareness is nonjudgmental, curious, and open to whatever appears in consciousness. It is important to point out that there is a difference between being nonjudgmental and not making judgements. Doctors need to make judgements, to choose between this or that antibiotic, or to start a new medication or not. Being nonjudgmental means giving space for whatever comes up in consciousness to be seen as it is before deciding either on its utility or its lack of usefulness. For example, when a physician working in an emergency room sees that the triage nurse has written on a patient's chart the reason for presentation as "requesting a prescription for fibromyalgia pain flare-up," a common set of prejudgments and negative stereotypes (specific emotions and thoughts) about the patient may appear in the physician's mind. Being nonjudgmental in this case does not mean not having negative thoughts and emotions but rather recognizing them as thoughts and emotions that arise (often unbidden) in consciousness and neither accepting them as true nor rejecting them as incorrect but rather being aware of them as sources of information to be tested and reassessed. The mindful physician still has unwanted thoughts and feelings that emerge (such as negative prejudgments), but it is what they then do, or do not do, with these prejudgments that makes all the difference.

Learning how to best approach complex medical issues is the raison d'être of the MMP course. We have found that the mindful doctor needs to be able to hold three aspects of conscious experience in awareness at the same time. First is the capacity to be aware, in a nonjudgmental way, of thoughts, physical sensations, and emotions from moment to moment. Second is an awareness of the whole person, the patient, who brings with them a problem they hope to have solved. Third is an awareness of the context in which the interaction is taking place, including the disease process that is manifesting in their patient, what is currently known and not yet known about pathophysiology, as well as evidence-based guidelines, protocols, and interventions, and how these may fit or not fit in with the particular person in front of them. Medical education has done well with ensuring the last of these, the awareness of disease processes, because they are easily standardized and measured in exams. The first two, mindful self-awareness and awareness of the patient, have increasingly been recognized as important [4, 5]. While we agree that these efforts can be helpful, we have found that medical students are less interested in learning mindfulness for its own intrinsic value and rather become more interested when the focus is on learning that directly connects to them becoming better doctors.

Mindful Clinical Congruence and the Good Doctor

We have coined the term mindful clinical congruence as the overall purpose of our teaching. The term congruence, from the work of Virginia Satir [6], refers to awareness of self, awareness of the other, and awareness of the context and is the three-pronged focus of the mindfulness that we teach. We have taught mindful congruence specifically as applied in a clinical context. Because the connection to learning to be a good doctor is made multiple times in each class, mindfulness skills become a means to a clear and universally agreed upon end. (Would anyone argue against learning to be a good doctor?) Therefore, teaching mindfulness skills such as focused attention is not about how to be a "mindful meditator" but rather is an essential skill in learning to be a good doctor. Is being able to focus on what the patient is saying, not saying, and how they are acting and reacting for at least 10 minutes at a time a skill that doctors should develop? If the answer is yes, then the question "Can you hold your attention for even 2 minutes at a time?" becomes one that captures students' interest and curiosity (see Chap. 3, Class 1). The goal is not to teach students how to be "good meditators" or how to psychoanalyze themselves and their patients, but rather is to have them learn what it takes to be a good clinician. Framed in this way, students are motivated to test themselves, for example, to see how well they can listen to others while being distracted first by their own cellphones and then by their own thoughts, emotions, and physical sensations. We think it is critically important to not only have students see for themselves how difficult it is to bring awareness to the three domains of being a good doctor but to give them hands-on practice with improving their capacities in class. We have created this mandatory pre-clerkship course to help give students practical skills they will practice together with us in class, to help them be the kind of doctor – attentive, respectful, and knowledgeable – that we all aspire to be.

Healing and Resilience

However, learning these skills is not just good for the patients our students will care for. It is also beneficial to their own well-being. We are teaching them skills that will help them do a better job of diagnosing and treating disease and facilitating healing in their patients. Healing is a move toward integrity and wholeness within the patient that can be facilitated by a healthcare practitioner. Healing is a two-way process. As Balfour Mount, one of the original promoters of this idea, has expressed it, "healing begets healing" [7]. When I as a physician have a healing interaction with my patient, it is not just the patient who experiences a move toward integrity and wholeness – I do too. We teach our students and have them experience that deep listening and relating is not a danger to be protected against but the key to rewarding practice and their most potent resource in promoting resilience and avoiding burnout.

Timing and How This Course Fits into a Healing Curriculum

The MMP course is taught at the end of the second year immediately prior to the beginning of clerkship. We believe that this timing is crucial. At this point in medical school, students are increasingly anxious about clerkship and are open to learning whatever will help them to be successful. Earlier in the curriculum we believe that students would have a harder time seeing the relevance of the course and later it would be difficult to teach it with the time constraints and preoccupations of clerkship overwhelming their attention. The 6 months prior to the major transition to intense clinical care is a hiatus period in which students are very open to learning what we have to teach.

That being said, we do prepare for and reinforce these lessons with sessions in the first, third, and fourth years. On the first day of medical school, we teach a class on healing and professionalism. Our aim in this, and in subsequent sessions in the first year, is to stress the importance of deep relating in the practice of medicine. At the end of the first year, we lead an interactive session with the whole class in which they reflect on the successes and challenges of the first year and what may help as they move into the second year. It is at this point that we introduce the idea of MMP and the course that we will teach in the second year. In the third year we work with students in the Simulation Centre, where they practice being mindfully congruent in dealing with stressful and conflictual clinical situations. In the fourth year, we return to the Simulation Centre, focusing on clinical interactions that the students themselves found challenging. We also conduct a whole class full-day session on clinical judgment that synthesizes what we have taught them and its relevance as they move forward to residency. One way that we have conceptualized our approach over the 4 years of medical school is as follows:

- *First year – Inspiration*: We attempt to keep alive and grow the spirit of caring that most students bring with them when starting medical school.
- *Second year – Preparation*: The MMP course prepares students for the challenges of intense clinical care.
- *Third year – Application*: We attempt to remind students of what they have learned about clinical relationships in the first 2 years and re-enforce its application in day-to-day clinical care.
- *Fourth year – Transition*: We target what they have learned to the specific challenges of residency and independent clinical practice.

We see this progression of teaching in the 4 years as a healing curriculum aimed at producing physicians who synergize technical competence and human caring to provide the best care to their patients. We taught elements of this curriculum in the past but have found that since introducing the MMP course, the overall effect of our teaching has markedly increased with this powerful course playing a pivotal role in the students' transition to effective clinical care.

References

1. Hutchinson TA. Whole person care: a new paradigm for the 21st century. New York: Springer Science+Business Media, LLC; 2011.
2. Hutchinson TA. Whole person care: transforming healthcare. Switzerland: Springer International Publishing; 2017.
3. Rizo CA, Jadad AR, Enkin M. What's a good doctor and how do you make one? BMJ. 2002;325:711. https://doi.org/10.1136/bmj.325.7366.711.
4. Dobkin PL, Hassed CS. Mindful medical practitioners: a guide for clinicians and educators. Switzerland: Springer; 2016.
5. Epstein R. Attending: medicine, mindfulness, and humanity. New York: Simon & Schuster, Inc; 2017.
6. Satir V, Banmen J, Gerber J, Gomori M. Congruence. In: The Satir model: family therapy and beyond. Palo Alto: Science and behavior books; 1991. p. 65–84.
7. Mount B, Kearney M. Healing and palliative care: charting our way forward. Palliat Med. 2003;17(8):657–8.

Chapter 2
Whole Person Teaching and Learning

Stephen Liben

Doing + Mindful Awareness = Learning

You do. You bring a specific type (mindful) of attention to the physical sensations, emotions, and thoughts of your lived experience as it is happening. Afterward, you bring mindful awareness to reflect on the experience. You see what worked and what did not work, and you create a story to explain what happened. You do it again, this time modifying your actions based on conclusions from past experience. Again, you bring mindful awareness to what happens both during and after the experience. You learn.

Mindful Teaching/Mindful Teacher

Mindful medical practice (MMP) students practice bringing their attention to what they are sensing, feeling, and thinking both while they are experiencing in the moment, and afterward, as sources of information from which clinical decisions can be made. Paying attention in a particular way, open to whatever appears, nonjudgmentally, and from moment to moment, is the action that cultivates the emergence of a specific type of awareness, called mindfulness. Paying attention in a particular way is what mindful meditation is. Mindfulness meditations, also referred to as guided awareness practice(s) (GAP) in this course, are one way to practice having mindful awareness emerge more often outside of formal meditation periods and are embedded as a core practice within each MMP class. A GAP is simple to understand cognitively (e.g., "bringing attention to the sensation of the breath…"); however, as students quickly see for themselves, it is not easy. Unlike other class exercises such as narrative writing or dyad discussions, in meditation exercises, the teacher is always an active participant. We have found that the only way to authentically lead a GAP is for the teacher to engage completely in the activity themselves

© Springer Nature Switzerland AG 2020
S. Liben, T. A. Hutchinson, *MD Aware*,
https://doi.org/10.1007/978-3-030-22430-1_2

from moment to moment. The tone of voice, the pacing of words, and the silences all emerge from the teacher's unscripted but well-practiced lived experience of their own practice.

Show, Don't Tell

An essential aspect of learning in MMP is that students are not explicitly told what they need to learn. Rather the topic is introduced and questions are asked to raise interest. For example, in Class 1 (Chap. 3), rather than explaining the limits of visual change perception as a concept, students are challenged to see for themselves if they can spot the change in a brief video clip of an otherwise stable scene. When they have the experience of not being able to perceive the visual changes at first (but once pointed out the change becomes impossible to miss), they "see" for themselves, rather than simply and less effectively having been told the learning point. Each class is structured as a sequence of group and individual experiences. Each new experience/activity is introduced and outlined, but not overly explained, so that students are not "told" in advance what they should be learning. Once students have had the particular learning experience, they are then invited to express (sometimes in dyads and other times as a large group) what they noticed. As they hear what other students have to say about their experience, the shared aspects of the learning experience naturally emerge. For example, rather than having the teacher explain before the GAP how common it is for the mind to wander off the sensation of the breath, students get to experience for themselves what happens when they try to keep their attention focused on their breath and then they see how their own experience is shared with others. Another way of stating this teaching method is to "show, don't tell."

Keeping It Personal

MMP is based on students experiencing *for themselves, in the classroom,* what is going on in the three domains of consciousness, namely, what they are experiencing from moment to moment as physical sensations, emotions, and thoughts. For example, in Class 6 (Chap. 8), Responding to Suffering, students engage in activities that explore what they have found to be both helpful and unhelpful when they themselves have suffered (e.g., a loss or a disappointment) that resulted from either getting what they did not want or not getting what they did want. The key element here is that students are encouraged to keep their attention on what **they themselves** are sensing, feeling, and thinking and about what is going on **for them**, right now, in this moment in class. By anchoring learning to what they themselves are experiencing, the tendency to judge, project, and overintellectualize the unknown experiences of others is reduced, and authenticity and the possibilities for learning something new about oneself are increased.

Learning "Made to Stick"

When we created MMP, we asked ourselves what we could easily bring to mind, even many years later, from all the talks we have heard or courses we ourselves have taken over the years. You may ask yourself the same question, and then see if the remembered idea included one or more of the six elements of "sticky ideas" – ideas that are simple, unexpected, concrete, credible, evoke emotion, and are told as a story. This is what Chip and Dan Heath described in their 2007 book *Made to Stick: Why Some Ideas Survive and Others Die* [1].

The first of these elements is simplicity. Ideas that are simple can be expressed in just a few words, such as the objective in Class 1 to recognize the limits of attention. The idea that an individual's ability to pay attention is finite and that we switch back and forth between competing attentional tasks rather than divide our attention into discrete separate units is simple to state but is not a "sticky" idea in and of itself. What makes the idea of limits to attention sticky in the first class is that we surprise students when we unexpectedly (the second aspect of sticky ideas) challenge them to prove us wrong (students love being challenged to prove us wrong!). We ask them to point out what changes in a brief video clip of an otherwise stable scene where only one thing changes over the course of 11 seconds. The "gradual change test" [2] is very difficult to notice at first, and to date no student has spotted the visual scene change until it has been pointed out to them. The instructions to the video are simple and we challenge students, "I bet you won't be able to spot the change." They then avidly watch the video and are invariably frustrated when they fail to notice what changes. Having had the experience of missing something that in retrospect looks impossible not to notice, the now sticky idea that "attention is limited" is easy to recall when coupled with feelings of frustration and surprise. The learning point becomes "sticky" because it has the elements of being simple, unexpected, and evoking emotion (third sticky element). The limits of attention are then reinforced in the concrete (fourth sticky element) hands-on "dyad cellphone exercise" later on in the same class, when students are asked to talk about something interesting to them while their partner is trying to both interact with their cellphone (social media, emails, etc.) and, at the same time, listen to their partner's story. This exercise is both unexpected (students are surprised when asked to interact with social media in class) and a concrete hands-on experience, illustrating the simple point that listening to someone with either full or partial attention is a choice that makes a difference to both the speaker and listener.

A good example of taking an otherwise sterile (not sticky) concept and bringing it to life, making it sticky, is how the Virginia Satir stances are brought from being *not known* before the course, to being *known* after they see the stances drawn on the whiteboard and explained in Class 2 (Chap. 4), to being *realized* when we have the students act out each stance in the role play in Class 4 (Chap. 6). In their end-of-course reflective essay, students often remark on how it was only in Class 4, after actively role playing the Satir stances in relation to the mock patient-doctor encounter, that they really understood how the stances could be useful to them clinically. The idea of the stances was credible (fifth sticky element) and known after they were explained in Class 2, but only after they were concretely embodied in Class 4 did students realize their practical usefulness and significance.

Stories, the sixth sticky element, are used in two ways to make learning stick. Firstly, stories are integrated into the formal MMP curriculum. For example, in Class 3 (Chap. 5) students watch the documentary short film "Just a Routine Operation" in which the husband tells the story of how his wife died in what should have been a routine operation [3]. The film includes a reenactment of what likely happened in the operating room that demonstrates a cascade of communication errors resulting in his young wife's completely unexpected brain death. The importance of communication and situational awareness in clinical settings is emotively brought out in the story that the bereaved husband narrates. The story of his wife's death transforms what could have been an otherwise arid set of learning points (e.g., the importance of communication and situational awareness) into a hard-to-forget sticky lesson on how and why things can go very wrong even with well-intentioned, experienced clinicians. As they watch the simulated operating room disaster unfold, students pay full attention to the video that is concrete, credible, and emotional, and afterward they are able to easily connect the involved professionals to specific Satir stances.

Personal stories are also used by MMP teachers informally on a spontaneous "prn" basis to illustrate ideas at different points in the course. These personal stories are ones that have been experienced by the teacher themselves and thus cannot be formalized into the course curriculum as each teacher needs to find their own authentic story to fit the relevant learning point. For example, in Class 7 (Chap. 9), each teacher needs to illustrate the iceberg model as it pertains to something going on for them personally in their own life. While teachers may pick the same issue to construct their iceberg, such as what their longings, perceptions, expectations, and emotions are in relation to teaching the MMP course itself, the specifics of each teacher's iceberg will be their own. The teacher's story of their iceberg is highly personal, and when used to illustrate how an iceberg model can be created, students are attentive because they can see and hear the embodied authentic and sometimes emotional effort being made by the teacher. Other examples are times when the teacher will have a story "at the ready" to illustrate a concept such as when demonstrating the progression from not knowing, to knowing, to realizing, and to actualizing in Class 7. A personal example that the coauthor (SL) has used is to describe a moment when he and his family are visiting his mother who lives in another country. On the first day of the visit, when he is not even really hungry, he opens her refrigerator door to see what he might eat. Unaware that his mother is standing a few feet behind him, he hears her start to list out loud each of the things she bought for him that she knows he likes. His initial reaction is one of surprise and irritation with her as he unconsciously finds himself reverting to his 12-year-old child self who felt controlled by her. He is aware of the felt physical sensation of his jaw clenching and the emotion of irritation that emerges unbidden and unwanted. He is then aware of the as yet unspoken thought his 12-year-old child self might answer back with: "I can see for myself what is in the fridge, Ma!" What follows is a moment of pausing that includes awareness of his reactivity and how he has played out this same scenario in the same way countless times in the past. In the pause he sees that there are other possibilities as his awareness now includes the transience of both their lives and the underlying intention of his mother who bought the food as an expression of love for him and his family. To his mother in that moment he says simply and lovingly, "Thank you, mom." The coauthor (SL) uses this as an example of knowing, as we all learn by about age 10 that we all will die one day, yet we may not fully "realize" the universality of death until we have our own close call with possible death such as after a car accident or new diagnosis. Even having had realizations of our own and everyone's finitude, we do not necessarily embody and actualize that knowledge as we continue to think and act as if those we love will always be there the next day. Actualizing that we all will die, and that everyone dies, would mean acting knowing that every word we say to those we love might be the last. In that moment, standing at the open door to his mother's refrigerator, the adult son responded (rather than reacted) out of that actualization.

While stories can be very helpful, the risk in using personal stories is that the teacher might unconsciously be telling a story for the wrong reasons and inadvertently deflect the focus of attention away from the students' own experiences. Unhelpful stories are those that go on too long, are not related directly to the material at hand, and have the effect of showing off and ego gratifying the storyteller themselves. We find that stories should be used like antibiotics, only when the benefit to risk ratio is high, in just the right dose, and sparingly.

The MMP Teacher: Creating "Wait, But Why?" Moments

What knowledge, skills, and attitudes does it take to teach MMP? The origin of the word "teacher," from the old English word to "show" or "point out," is a good description of the MMP teacher who is tasked with pointing things out, rather than telling or lecturing to students. In practice, pointing out is distinct from telling and is the reason we have specifically avoided using audiovisual slides in this course. One benefit of prepared teaching slides is that teachers can ensure that all students are exposed to (but do not necessarily learn) the same "material." However, we do not think that exposure to information, in this age when handheld devices are open portals to almost everything that has ever been written, should be the reason for gathering students together in class. Rather, the purpose of teaching is to bring knowledge, skills, and attitudes through the stages of learning from what is not known, through knowing, then realizing, to then actualizing into daily life. We have found that the disadvantages far outweigh the possible benefits of pre-prepared teaching slides in MMP. Once slides are projected onto a screen, an unspoken but powerful dynamic is set in motion. Teachers then become lecturers telling students content that they are expert in, with little room for either questioning or dissenting. Students enter into a passive observer "watching" mode of being that feels very comfortable, familiar, and non-threatening. So what is wrong with feeling good and being completely comfortable in the knowledge that you will not be threatened with being asked to share your thoughts? There is nothing inherently wrong with feeling such comfort, but it is also not the most conducive to learning, particularly if the learning involves challenging concepts you thought you already knew. For example, say you had learned, and you still believe, that compassion and empathy are inherent rather than learnable traits and that you "either have them or you don't." If a lecturer then tells you otherwise that compassion is the result of specific factors many of which are in each person's locus of control, then what is your motivation to change what you had previously thought to be true? Why should you believe this new and contradictory idea even if it is from an "expert"? How does real learning take place and how often have you yourself changed what you thought simply based on hearing, even an expertly stated, contrary opinion? When what we thought we knew is challenged or when we hear something that we did not even know we did not know, there is a moment of cognitive dissonance, a "wait, but why?" moment. If the teacher has challenged the preconception of the student in just the right way, nonjudgmentally (i.e., mindfully), then "wait, but why?" is evoked in the student. In the first part of "wait, but why," the "wait…," is the element of surprise, the moment of cognitive dissonance, the feeling of "not being comfortable." This being slightly uncomfortable is energy that sharpens attention that then evolves into curiosity, the "…but why." The state of "…but why" is the ideal condition – curious, open, and energized by being slightly uncomfortable – and is where learning happens.

Are we advocating for the creation of class experiences that might, at times, make some students slightly uncomfortable? Indeed, we are. We find that a small measure of discomfort, not knowing exactly what we will be coming up next in class and what may be asked of the student, is the ideal condition for learning to happen. These conditions of just the correct amount of discomfort and unpredictability are unstable as they are subject to what is going on with students from moment to moment in class. The teacher's task is to make frequent small adjustments to the tone of the class, to keep the tension balanced between feeling comfortable enough to create trust with the counterpoint of unpredictability that keeps students' attention focused. Much like tuning the strings of a guitar, there is a balance point of tension that is just right for staying in tune. This balance point is inherently unstable as it will change with both the teacher and the individual student's attention and comfort/discomfort level within any particular activity. The teacher's task is subtle and a bit of a dance to keep readjusting the balance point of tension to changing conditions. Do one or two students in the group appear withdrawn or bored? Perhaps this is the time to invite them to share what they are thinking on the topic being addressed. Is another student talking too much and unaware of how their peers are nonverbally but clearly reacting negatively? Maybe this is the time to gently thank the talkative student and ask for the thoughts of others who have not yet spoken.

The Teacher: Great Faith, Great Doubt, and Great Effort

Taken from the conditions for practice in Zen Buddhism, great faith, great doubt, and great effort are requisites for teaching MMP. Great faith describes the teacher's need to have faith that what they are bringing to the MMP class is going to be enough and that they themselves are enough. The teacher enters the class and sits on a chair in the circle with no difference between their seat and any of the students' seats and no raised platform to stand on or podium to stand behind. Teachers are challenged to hold the attention for almost 2 hours of 20 high-achieving, skeptical, science-oriented students, many of whom have stereotype-based incorrect ideas of what the course is about (e.g., "it's about not thinking" or "it's about relaxing or mental health") and who come from very diverse backgrounds, cultures, and belief systems. What the teacher has in hand for these 2 hours is one sheet of paper with an outline of concepts and activities. The MMP teacher needs to walk into each class with the faith that what they have with them is enough and that together with the students, learning will happen. Each of the seven classes and each time a class is taught is both the same and never the same. The broad outline of what will happen and the learning objectives for each class are clear; the "what" to do is outlined on the one-page class summary, while the "how" the class will evolve is never the same. The MMP teacher is like the experienced sailor who has sailed before, knows the boat can handle the sea, and has a navigation chart in hand to show the way. What the sailor does not know is what the weather will be like. He or she knows where to go, how to get there, and what could come up, but what will actually occur in the form of either helpful winds or new obstacles along the way remains unknown until it happens. What the sailor and the MMP teacher need is faith to remain open and know they can handle whatever comes up. Some classes go well with minimal interventions by the teacher, while at other times a class may require more involvement in maintaining students' attention.

Great doubt is required, as well. The MMP teacher needs to let go of their own preconceptions of how the class "should happen." Great doubt is allowing what needs to come up in class to come up, including the possibility that the teacher themselves may be, or feel to be, challenged and doubted. The teacher needs to have the capacity to be resilient and flexible as the same material will not be accepted by every student in the same way. The key to holding this doubt is the awareness that nothing of what is happening is personal, very little if anything is about the teacher themselves. Students will react or respond based on their history and state at the time, all of which is unknowable by the teacher and often by the students themselves.

Great effort refers not so much to the necessary effort that starts with teacher training in observing the course, then co-teaching with an experienced teacher, and then mentally rehearsing days before each class they will teach by themselves. Great effort rather refers to the effort to reopen the mind and heart to why they are teaching this course, despite the hardships, internal and external obstacles, and lack of external recognition that may be the case. Great effort comes naturally out of great faith and doubt in seeing for yourself the transformational learning that happens in class when the right conditions are created. For example, hearing a student say "I thought I knew what was important in my life until we did the decreasing length of time exercise that forced me to look at my life again with new eyes" is a great motivator for the teacher to maintain the extra effort that is required when, at moments, both the students and teacher are less inspired.

Course Time and Timing

We purposively set up our curriculum to teach three MMP classes at the same time each week (Friday mornings) in three classrooms physically next to each other. With this set up, three sets of 20 students can be taught simultaneously each week for the 7 weeks of the course. This allows for the teaching of 60 students per 7-week course block and for a total of 180 students over a 6-month period. We created a 3-hour time block that is reserved just for MMP each Friday morning from 9:00–12:00. This 3-hour time period is one where both students and MMP teachers have no other obligations. Teachers arrive at least 30 minutes (and often even 60 minutes) before each class to set up the rooms (removing tables, adding or subtracting chairs, placing chairs in a circle) and ensure audiovisual equipment, pens, paper pads, and markers are ready. Because all three classes start at the same time in the same location, teachers also support each other in setting up their rooms and can help each other troubleshoot audiovisual issues or questions about a particular class exercise. Because each MMP class is 90–120 minutes in duration, this leaves time for both after-class individual student- or teacher-initiated conversations as well as for a post-class teacher-only debrief.

Teacher Debriefing

We view the post-class teacher debrief as an essential support for MMP teachers and as critical for their own teaching expertise development. The teacher debrief is structured so that successive class activities are reviewed by each teacher in turn, to reflect upon what went well and what did not go so well with each activity and for each teacher. The conversation is not about what should be changed in the curriculum, but rather it is an opportunity to discuss how different teachers handle the type of issues that come up (such as the "low energy" or "high energy" group of students or the "difficult" student) or to share the different nuances that more experienced teachers have learned for particular exercises. The emotional support that emerges is as important as the content aspect (hearing how other teachers approach the same exercises) of these debriefs. The teacher debriefs also serve as self- and other-monitoring for authenticity: Are the debriefs themselves co-led as embodied whole person teaching and learning? Are there opportunities for personal growth for the teachers themselves as the three-person small group of teachers helps each other see possible personal blind spots such as a "blaming the student" (Satir) stance? How is the teachers' debrief like and not like the MMP classes themselves? These are the kinds of questions that can emerge in teacher debriefs and are part of what helps each teacher to also remain a learner themselves.

The Right Space

The wise gardener knows that when preparing the garden, good soil, protection from the elements, and careful cultivation are absolutely necessary but not sufficient in and of themselves for plants to grow. Once the garden has been carefully set up, the gardener does not "make" plants grow but rather watches as growth unfolds from the complex interaction of the elements with the potential already present in the seeds. In a similar way, the physical structure of the classroom is an essential but not sufficient condition for MMP small group learning. The right space for MMP small group learning is a physical classroom that removes obstacles that would otherwise detract from students' capacity to learn.

While the amount of administrative course support may vary, the minimal essential conditions required to teach effectively are ultimately the responsibility of the MMP teacher. The MMP teacher will need to ensure the class is set up correctly each time, which means getting to class early enough to have time to set up the circle of chairs, bring in extra chairs, or remove unneeded chairs. Additionally, tables may need to be removed from the room in order to create an open space for the circle of chairs, and audiovisual equipment for Classes 1 and 3 needs to be set up in advance to ensure they will run as needed, at the correct volume and at the exact time they are needed.

In the same way the MMP teacher does not "role model" but rather embodies a mindful clinician-teacher, the physical classroom of a simple circle of chairs with everyone facing the center embodies the values of inclusivity and equality (no implied hierarchy in seating positions) and fairness (no one, the teacher themselves included, gets to hide behind a physical structure). The classroom requirements for MMP are simple and are critically important to not waiver from when the inevitable request to modify them is made due to the reality of space limitations in most medical schools. For example, requests may be made to teach MMP in groups larger than the maximum of 25 students, or to use an auditorium instead of a small classroom, or to use a room with immovable desks and chairs fixed to the floor. The good gardener knows that without water all other efforts to grow plants would be futile in the same way that the MMP teacher knows what is essential and what is optional for teaching. What follows is a list of the essential elements for the MMP classroom.

Essential Classroom Requirements

1. Classroom sized to hold 10–25 students.

   – Less than 10 students and the group dynamic shifts away from what the MMP course as outlined in this book was structured for. There are other ways of teaching smaller groups, but the class exercises in MMP would need to be modified for groups smaller than 10 students.
   – More than 25 students and the circle created becomes too large to maintain the level of immediacy and intimacy that proximity facilitates.

2. Doors that can close off the room from outside sounds.
3. Inside-facing walls opaque or semi opaque to outside viewers.
4. Chairs on rollers or movable chairs so that the teacher can ensure that there is only one chair per student with no extra empty chairs in the room before each class begins. Extra chairs (for students who unexpectedly did not attend) are removed by the teacher just before the class in order to create a closed circle with no empty gaps.
5. A white board with markers, or blackboard with chalk, or a large poster board with removable sheets of paper and markers.
6. The capacity to show a video with audio for Classes 1 and 3.

Nonessential Classroom Requirements

1. Outside-facing windows for natural rather than artificial light.
2. If more than one class is being taught at a time (we teach three classes simultaneously with three teachers, each with 20 students per class), then it is ideal to have the three classrooms be very close to each other. In this way, teachers are in close proximity to each other both for the unexpected that may arise and for coordinating the post-class teacher debrief.

Distractions to Leave Out of the Classroom

1. Cellphones, laptops, and notebooks are useful in some settings but not in an MMP small group where they serve as distractions. If students object to not being able to take notes during class, we assure them that all potentially testable didactic points in the class have been summarized in study notes that are available to them throughout the course.
2. Pre-prepared audiovisual slides and handouts of illustrations and diagrams are not used in MMP. Instead, all drawings are illustrated by hand at the time they are needed. Having the MMP teacher draw out, markers in hand, all the

required diagrams (e.g., triangle of attention) feels something like the difference between listening to pre-recorded music versus being present at a live performance. The live performance is always technically imperfect compared with studio-recorded music, and yet while its specific qualitative advantage may be ineffable, it has an aliveness, a creativeness that translates into a felt energy. We feel that there is a "live performance" aspect to all good teaching. A good teacher, like a good theater actor or musician, needs to prepare in advance by studying the material, prepare mentally to be fully present and alive to those in the shared space, and project interest and enthusiasm.

Small Group Teaching and Learning

There are often felt differences between student small groups from year to year, as some groups seem more talkative or open than others, dependent on individual personalities, backgrounds, and life experiences. There are also many common issues that come up repeatedly from small group to small group. Some of the recurring issues and ways we have found to address them are as follows.

The Reluctant Student

Possible reasons for a student not being open to participate include an acute personal crisis (e.g., parental illness), mental health issue such as depression or anxiety, shyness, fear of public embarrassment, or resistance to what they perceive the class and course to be about (as opposed to its actual learning objectives). The teacher needs to be mindful and first skillfully assess why the student does not participate in group discussions or other activities such as writing exercises. Clues to the reasons are often evident in the student's nonverbal in-class behavior. Is the student looking particularly sad and/or anxious? If so, and if this is noticed during more than one class, then it might be helpful to speak to the student privately after class to gently inquire, "Is there something stopping you from more fully participating?" Is the student behaving in ways that suggest resistance to the course material or to a mistaken idea that the course is about "wellness" and should be optional? If so, then asking that student what he or she thinks the course is about and allowing them to state their objections and then have others in the class help answer questions and possible misunderstandings might be helpful. The teacher may need to reframe that the course is about essential clinical skills, such as how to best manage the angry or resistant patient (or colleague), and then see if they agree that these are skills worth exploring.

The Overenthusiastic Student

A student may be talking a lot and not leaving enough space for others to participate in group discussions. Small group teaching skills are helpful here including first acknowledging the student ("Thank you offering your thoughts.") and then redirecting to others in the group ("I wonder if we might hear from those who have not yet had the opportunity to speak?"). At other times there may be students in the class who have some prior experience with mindfulness meditation, and they may either resist class activities with an attitude of "That's not how I learned to do this" or, alternatively, they may try to convince and "sell" (i.e., to tell, and not show) the value of mindfulness practices to the other students. Acknowledging each student, seeing and not judging them, and at the same time gently redirecting to what others are experiencing are small group teaching skills that are essential for MMP teachers.

The Disruptive Student

Students may disrupt class activities by being passive-aggressive or aggressive in different ways. During meditation exercises the disruptive student may subtly slouch back in their chair during instructions to find a position of wakeful alertness and then tap their foot during the brief periods of silent meditation. Other ways to be disruptive include students who argue and disagree on every learning point being brought out. The MMP teacher will need to be particularly mindful themselves to not become reactive and inadvertently add to the student's disruptive behavior. "What might be helpful now?" is a helpful question for the teacher to consider in the moment. Is this behavior that needs to be addressed immediately and is it a recurring pattern, or is better to wait to see if it recurs? Is this behavior something to discuss in group discussion during class or alternatively with the individual student after class? We suggest not waiting too long to address this type of behavior as it can escalate over time and then negatively impact the learning experience of other students.

The Depressed or Anxious Student

While students with depression or anxiety or both may manifest with any of the above behaviors, we have found that the depth of the issue often only becomes apparent in an after-class one-on-one private conversation that was either student- or teacher-initiated. A teacher simply privately asking a student of concern, "How are you doing?" especially if said empathically, may evoke admissions of thoughts of suicide or other significant mental health issues that may require immediate medical intervention by the MMP teacher. We have outlined pathways for our teachers to access immediate local student mental health services if required, and we recommend that all MMP teachers have knowledge of their local resources for students in need.

The Late or Leaving Early Student

During the first class, students are given explicit instructions that they must be in the classroom before the door closes at the start of each class and that they will not be allowed into the classroom late and will then be considered to have missed that day's class. There are also students who ask to leave a class early for some other activity they have scheduled before the 2-hour period of the class would be completed. Students may complain that it is "not fair" to be considered absent if they are "only 1 minute late for a class." We have found that these issues are worthy of discussion in class, but not compromise, should they come up. We understand and agree with students that "buses may be late" and "weather can be an unpredictable factor." We ask students to consider that we as teachers also have these same issues to contend with and we plan for them so that we will not be late if we miss a bus or are caught in traffic. We also explore the idea that they will be expected to arrive on time for all their clinical activities such as arriving to relieve a colleague who worked overnight in the emergency room, scrubbing into an operating room, or arriving for a clinic that has patients waiting to see them. We ask them to consider arriving early enough to have more than enough time to spare and to use that time to either do some work or read or simply be still for a few minutes before class begins. We ask students who self-identify as "I'm always late or just in time" to come in even extra early one morning and see what they notice (particularly in their physical sensations) when they arrive early versus when they arrive "just in time." We similarly do not allow any student to leave early for another activity and we may point out that we ourselves have also committed to the full 2 hours. Students may not agree about many aspects of their medical education or about the importance of, for example, a subject such as anatomy if they already know they want to be a psychiatrist, and yet the standards of medical education are not based primarily on student preferences. If an MMP class is missed, then there is an imperfect but workable system in place to "make up" a missed class that will be discussed in the 11th chapter (see Chap. 11: Mindful Medical Practice and the Good Doctor).

The Taking Many Breaks During Class Student

In the 90–120-minute class, there are no scheduled breaks for the bathroom. In Class 1 we state that students may leave to briefly use the bathroom as they are expected to be adult learners. There are rare occasions when one or more students leave repeatedly and thus disrupt the class activities. When this occurs, one way to address the issue is to bring up in class that the teacher has noticed the disruption that this leaving creates and could remind students that staying in a room for 90 minutes without taking a break is well within the norms expected within clinical practice. If there are individual students with specific health or other issues who have difficulty, then this could be addressed after class in a one-on-one private interview.

Learning to Stay: Contemplative Practices

We define contemplative practice as an activity in which conscious attention is intentionally focused for a pre-defined period of time on a mental object, either a physical sensation, an emotion, or a thought, and where attention is brought back as many times as needed when awareness of having moved off the object occurs. In MMP, contemplative practices include "body scans" and mindfulness of the breath as well as of other physical sensations (e.g., soles of the feet exercise). The most commonly used exercise is a seated GAP where the teacher first provides instruction on seated posture and then verbally guides the class as to where attention may be placed and what to do when attention has drifted off. Each teacher will have their unique way of guiding meditations, all with the intention of having students observe for themselves what comes up in their experience within these focused attention exercises. While most students are open to trying these activities as "experiments" some may express concerns such as:

- "I am not able to quiet my mind, I don't think I can do it." We might first ask the other students in the group who also had many thoughts to raise their hand (typically many students will raise their hand). We might then reflect that there is no need to quiet the mind and that is not the intention. Rather the goal, or intention, is to be aware of whatever physical sensations, emotions, or thoughts are occurring but that there is no right or wrong way to be. What matters is not *what* thoughts occur, neither their presence nor their content, but rather *that* they are occurring and can be noted and noticed within awareness.
- "I can't sit still, I just have to move." We might ask if this student is able to notice the physical sensations and thoughts associated with their "need to move." Can they move as little as possible and let that be ok? As long as the student is not disrupting others with their movements, then the "need to move" and even the movements themselves are simply to be noted and allowed as what is occurring now.
- "I refuse to follow the directions as you cannot tell me what to do if I don't want to" or "I don't like the way you give instructions as I learned to meditate another way." The teacher may point out that the instructions are suggestions being offered and are not commands to be obeyed. The teacher cannot know what each student is actually thinking in any case, and as long as the student does not

disrupt the possible learning experience of others, they are free to think whatever they like during the brief contemplative exercises.

For teachers, guiding these contemplative practices is not something that you can "fake it until you make it." Teachers need to have some prior practice in guiding groups and should have a base experience of meditation themselves for a period of time before teaching. How much prior experience and for how long are not known. What we do know is that a teacher guiding meditations needs to bring themselves to the practice in the moment with 100% authenticity. To guide a practice is to practice, and any inauthenticity is quickly detected by self and others. The tone and cadence of speech when guiding meditations is not a teacher "playing a role," but rather emerges as an in-the-moment, live, embodied expression of what the teacher themselves is experiencing from moment to moment.

References

1. Heath C, Heath D. Made to stick: why some ideas survive and others die. New York: Random House; 2007.
2. Simons DJ, Franconeri S, Reimer RL. Change blindness in the absence of a visual disruption. Perception. 2000;29(10):1143–54. https://doi.org/10.1068/p3104.
3. McClelland G, Smith MB. Just a routine operation: a critical discussion. J Perioper Pract. 2016;26(5):114–7.

Chapter 3
Class 1: Attention and Awareness

Stephen Liben

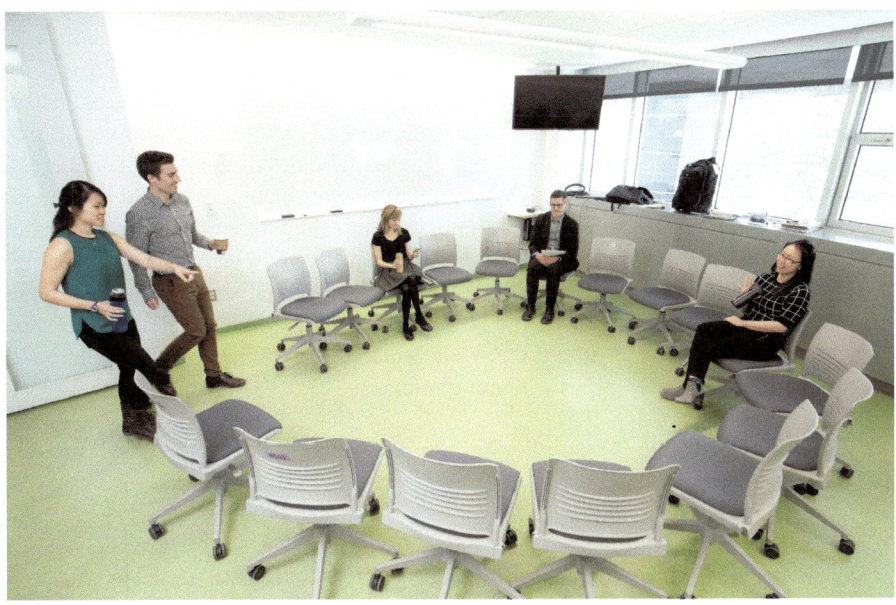

Fig. 3.1 Students entering MMP class for the first time

Overview

Students arrive for their first Mindful Medical Practice (MMP) class, coffee cups, water bottles, and cellphones in hand (Fig. 3.1). Many are talking to each other and/ or texting as they walk in. Some enter the class and have a look of surprise on their face when they see the chairs (with no desks or tables) facing each other in a circle.

© Springer Nature Switzerland AG 2020
S. Liben, T. A. Hutchinson, *MD Aware*,
https://doi.org/10.1007/978-3-030-22430-1_3

They may or may not make eye contact with the teacher as they choose their seat. They finally all arrive and are seated.

This first class of the course has its own specific challenges and opportunities for the teacher. Students will likely have heard about the MMP course from previous students, and they enter the class with their own individual preconceptions, some of which are accurate but many of which are incorrect assumptions about the purpose of the course. A challenge for the MMP teacher is to connect each class to essential clinical skills in communication and decision-making required of all clinicians. Some students erroneously believe that a course with "mindfulness" in the title is about "relaxing," while the reality is that MMP is designed to meet learning objectives essential for competent clinical care. The word "mindfulness" is often mistakenly used as a synonym for "thoughtfulness." While mindfulness includes thoughts (together with emotions and physical sensations), it is not *what* you are thinking, but rather an awareness *that* you are thinking.

Opportunities to explore and question what is being taught in class and why will come up repeatedly in this and future classes, and there will be many openings for the teacher to connect a class activity to an identified clinical skill. In this first class, the role of attention is explicitly explored, and the connection to care of patients is emphasized in different exercises that are intentionally stimulating and very different from sitting in a lecture hall listening to a PowerPoint presentation. Another task of the teacher in this first class is to have students see for themselves what is expected of them both in terms of the formal course curriculum (e.g., attendance, written essay, and exam) and the informal expectation that they will be called upon to think and contribute to class activities and conversations. The educational underpinning of the entire course is to provide the structure necessary for students to experience for themselves, instead of being passively lectured to, what they need to know to become knowledgeable caring resilient clinicians.

1. Introducing the MMP Class

> Good morning. We are going to begin by having you say your first and last name and then what your name means to you. You might want to say where the origin of your name came from, or perhaps what you have been told what your name (first or last) means. We'll start with whomever feels ready to speak....

Each student then takes about 1 minute to say something about what their name means to them. The exercise is complete when each student has spoken. The teacher may decide, based on their personal preference, whether to talk about the meaning of their own name.

The very first words spoken in class by the teacher are intentionally in the form of a question, asking students to reflect on the meaning of their name. We begin the course by asking a question to enact the concept that they will be asked to think and to reflect, rather than being given information or being told facts. What is implicit in this first interaction is the expectation that students are to be active participants rather than passive recipients of information. This structured self-reflection exercise is also an opportunity to build group cohesiveness, as students learn something new and personal about their classmates despite already having spent much time together over the previous two years.

After asking students to say their name and what it means to them, we have used two different ways to facilitate how they respond. One way is to have them speak sequentially one after another in the order in which they are seated. Going around the circle (either clockwise or counterclockwise) has the disadvantage of a decrease in the capacity to listen to others just before it is their turn to speak, as they focus their attention on rehearsing to themselves what they will say rather than listening to others. Once a student has spoken there is a further fall off of attention for those who are socially shy and are now feeling relieved that their turn in the spotlight is over. An alternate way to instruct students, rather than going sequentially around the circle, is to invite the first student that is ready to speak to do so and then continue with whomever is ready next to speak. In this less structured way of inviting students to speak when they are ready, they will be less sure when it will actually be their turn, and this uncertainty may help to sustain attention.

The group is then asked, "What do you think this course is about?" Responses are often along the lines of "to help us be relaxed," "to have us be calm in difficult situations," and "I don't understand what this course is about." Students should be allowed to express their preconceived ideas about the class, including incorrect negative concepts (e.g., "I don't see why I should be forced to meditate"). The teacher needs to walk a sensitive line between allowing what is thought and felt to be expressed, while additionally, when the timing is right, to gently but clearly correct misperceptions. For example, after a strongly worded objection is voiced such as "being forced to meditate," it can be pointed out that while there will be regular brief periods of guided awareness/meditation, during this time what each student actually does in their own mind remains up to them. As long as students sit quietly, no one is going to force them to think or not think anything in particular. If said with compassion and understanding by the teacher who is not surprised by these kinds of student objections and concerns, it can be reinforced that paying attention is an important clinical skill, and they are being offered to experience for themselves methods on how to focus and refocus attention that they may find helpful when faced with "real-life" challenging clinical situations. It can also be offered that this course is a unique opportunity for students to see for themselves the possible benefits of different contemplative practices in a small group setting with 7 weeks of continuity – a protected period of time that will be increasingly difficult to replicate as they advance in their medical careers. Students are encouraged to withhold judgments as to whether they like or do not like the various activities they will be practicing until they have had the full experience of the course. An analogy can be offered that it would take time before being able to judge whether an individual could play the piano or other musical instrument, and it would be unrealistic to predict a future pianist's musical potential after only the first few hours of practice.

The group is next asked, "Why is MMP offered at this time in the curriculum (just before clerkship)?" Students often correctly answer that the course is offered just before clerkship because they might not appreciate its relevance to clinical practice if it was offered in the first year of medical school. If offered later, during clerkship when intense clinical activity had begun, it would be difficult to create the needed time (protected from clinical responsibilities) that the course requires. The timing of the course is similar to preparing for what needs to be done before a canoe on a swiftly flowing river approaches a set of rapids. The time to practice safety maneuvers and review and rehearse what to do and not to do is in the calm water before the rough water of the rapids. Just before clerkship is analogous to the calm water, an ideal time to practice clinical skills that will be needed in the controlled and safe environment of the classroom.

The final question is then asked, "In what possible clinical scenarios might your capacity to pay attention be important?" By having students think through and artic-ulate situations where attentional capacity will be important (e.g., in a busy emer-gency department), they are more likely to internalize the learning objective that paying attention is an important clinical skill that is worth exploring than if they were told the same message in a didactic lecture.

2. Guided Awareness Practice

The teacher needs to have some prior personal experience both with meditation and with guiding specific types of meditations. This experience can be acquired as part of MMP teacher training (see Chap. 2: "Whole Person Teaching and Learning"). While it is not practical for every teacher to have extensive meditation and medita-tion guiding experience, it is also true that this is an especially embodied learning experience where the nonverbal aspects are as important as which words are used. What we have called a guided awareness practice (GAP) in the MMP course is a synonym for a specific type of guided meditation that uses the breath and body as attentional anchors. When the meditation is a sequential guide to bringing attention to specific and successive parts of the body, it is called a "body scan." When atten-tion is focused on the sensation of the breath at either the nose and mouth or in the rising and falling of the abdomen, it is a "breath meditation."

In this very first 5–7-minute GAP, the teacher takes time to set up a suggested body posture and then begins the guided meditation as a partial body scan, starting with bringing attention to the sensation of feet on the floor and ending with 2 min-utes of attention focused on the sensation of breathing as felt in the abdomen.

For many students this will be their first guided meditation experience, while others will have had previous experience with different types of meditation prac-tices. This first meditation has more verbal guidance by the teacher and less silence than will be the case as the course progresses, as verbal cues are most helpful when beginning to learn how to focus attention. Out of the 5–7 minute body scan from the feet to abdomen that segues to awareness of the breath, there should be about 3 minutes of silence left between the last words said aloud, "rest-ing attention on the sensation of the abdomen as it rises and falls with each breath," and the end of the meditation. After the first minute of silence, the teacher may choose to insert into the silence a brief verbal reminder/instruction that, "If you find your attention has drifted away from the breath onto a thought, that's okay. Gently bring your attention back to the sensation of the breath, and if this happens many times, then bring your attention back to the breath just that many times." The large group debrief begins when the GAP is concluded with words such as "When you are ready, open your eyes if they are closed and bring your attention from the sensation of your breath back to the class." The large group is then asked, "What did you notice?" Additional more directed questions may also be asked, such as "Was it easy or hard to follow the instructions?" and "Were you able to fully focus attention on the breath or was your attention carried away by thoughts?" In this first meditation debrief, a major role of the teacher is to normalize the many different possible responses. Normalizing what was noticed (such as feeling sleepy or distracted) is facilitated by the teacher commenting directly (e.g., by stating "that is quite common") or by asking who else in the group noticed a similar phenomenon to highlight the commonality of experience. Normalization of the many types of experiences in meditation is most powerful when it comes from the direct experiences of students rather than from teacher statements.

Some students will be more willing and comfortable to share their experience with the group than others, particularly at this early stage of the course. Typically, no more than 2–3 students will speak in response to the "What did you notice?" prompt. It may be wise not to require others to speak at this early point in the class, that is, not to "push" the shy or skeptical students. In subsequent classes there will be many opportunities for the teacher to encourage hearing from students who are less comfortable volunteering to share their experiences with the large group.

It can be expected that students will have a variety of reactions to the first GAP including:

- Enjoying and appreciating the experience
- Being unsure "what the point is"
- Finding it very challenging to follow the instructions and being lost in thought
- Mistakenly thinking that meditation is about "feeling relaxed"
- Being so unaware of their unawareness that they are convinced they easily maintained the focus of their attention on their breath, with no thoughts arising for the full duration of the exercise
- Not saying anything in the debrief as they may remain wary that what they say will be judged by the teacher and other students

In this first GAP exercise debrief, it is best for the teacher to avoid overcorrecting students who misunderstand the intention of the exercise and instead validate and redirect to what might be more helpful. For example, if a student states that this was a great "relaxation exercise" rather than an opportunity to practice paying attention in a certain way, the teacher might validate that "at times meditation may be relaxing" and also add that no matter what is noticed it is the noticing itself that is important. Should students offer an interpretation of their experience (e.g., "I felt relaxed"), the teacher may redirect them to investigate, "What specifically were you feeling in your body at that time?"

3. Change Blindness Video

Change blindness occurs when an observer is unable to notice a change in a visual stimulus. The phenomenon is best experienced rather than explained, and there are many video-based examples of change blindness that are widely available. We use a brief video of the changing of a rock into vegetation that is very difficult to notice on first viewing [1].

After watching the video, most if not all students will have failed to notice the visual change, and their comments often include finding reasons why they were not able to note the change despite prior prompting. For example, some students have said, "We should have been warned that it was going to be a slow transition." Others are surprised at how they were not able to track what in retrospect looks like a very obvious change. The point of the exercise is to have them experience for themselves that paying attention, even to one brief visual stimulus, while simple in theory, is not easy in practice. Being aware of all stimuli that present to the nervous system as an ongoing stream of changing sights, sounds, smells, tastes, and touches is beyond the capacity of any individual. The mind is not a passive receptacle for all incoming data; it processes information within its attentional limits and necessarily filters out what is deemed to be less important at any one time.

Students are then asked, "What are possible clinical correlates to this phenomenon?" This leads to a group discussion of clinical situations where attention is pulled in different directions. The many examples include the need to notice and then discern the relevance of a bedside cardiorespiratory monitor alarm and the need for increased attention when a patient is leaving the office and has "one more quick question before I go." (The so-called "doorknob question" is often what the patient is most worried about but was afraid to bring up earlier.)

In understanding that attentional capacity is inherently limited, it is important to think about the question: "If attention is so limited then what can be done to help improve attentional capacity?" Appreciating that the capacity to pay attention and notice change is limited, and that it is possible to practice how to focus and refocus attention within guided awareness exercises as a way to strengthen attentional capacity, is one of the main learning objectives of this class. Far from implying that students need to just "pay better attention to everything," this exercise also highlights the value and necessity of listening to others involved in patient care who can point out what any one person might have otherwise missed.

4. Four Minutes of Red Exercise

The following is an example of a playful way to introduce this exercise in focused attention: "This activity is effective only when done in complete silence. In addition to what we all understand is verbal silence is something called 'silence of the eyes,' where you intentionally do not make direct eye contact with others. When you are asked to start, and please not before then, your task will be to find and list on your paper as many red objects as you can see from inside this room. You are allowed to get up out of your chair and move around the room to look for more red objects, as long as you remain silent. The winner will be the student with the longest list. The winner might win a prize of a cup of coffee or a million dollars. Who knows?! Now, before we begin, are there any questions?"

The possibly that the student with the longest list might win a million dollars or a cup of coffee is said with body language that makes it clear that the prize is not to be taken seriously. The preferences of the teacher should dictate just how this exercise is introduced as the outrageously exaggerated million-dollar prize will not work for everyone's teaching style. If a student asks how they are to judge if something is "red enough" to add to their list, or if something might be considered pink and not red, the teacher might say that it is up to them to decide what is red and what is not red. "Remember to make your list as long as possible. Begin now!" If students begin talking at any point during the 4 minutes gently remind them of the importance of remaining silent for this exercise.

After 3–4 minutes have passed, ask students to silently return to their seats and count up the total number of red items on their list. The student with the greatest number of items, no matter what is on it in terms of what they labeled as red, is declared the "winner." We then ask the "winner" and two other students to each write their lists on the whiteboard (each student is given a different color marker). As a large group exercise, we then have the rest of the group compare their own lists with the ones written on the white board. We then ask, "What did you notice as you made your lists?" in addition to asking these possible additional questions:

- Were there more red items in the room than you first thought?
- Did you miss some red items? If you did miss some, does that surprise you?
- How did you decide what was "red enough" to add it to your list? How might the prize for the longest list influence what you decided was "red enough"?
- How might this process of selecting an item as "red or not" be relevant to clinical decision-making, such as when faced with a binary clinical decision like the need to do a lumbar puncture or not?

What students most often raise in discussion is that some of the items on the list of "what is red" were not considered "red enough" by everyone else to "count" as an item. This allows the teacher to raise the question of how decisions are made when situations are framed as "this or that" binary choices. While at first glance binary choices seem to be simple ones, a closer look reveals the arbitrariness of many binary decisions and at the same time demonstrates that when things are not clear (such as the difference between red and not red), then other factors, both conscious and unconscious, come into the decision-making process. What helped students determine that something that was "somewhere on the spectrum from pink to red" on first glance was then chosen to be "red enough" to ultimately be placed on their list? Did the reward based on having the greatest number of red items put some pressure on decision-making to tip any one decision towards "yes, indeed it's red enough to go on my list"? What would happen to decision-making if the stakes were truly a million dollars? How might a high reward or a large risk influence decision-making in so-called binary situations?

At this point in the conversation, some students may be thinking, "So what if binary choices are not as clear as at first seems?" Students can be asked, "How might the way you place your attention and make binary choices be clinically relevant in your medical decision-making with patients?" This is an opportunity for students to make the connection that binary choices, while often useful in practice, are rarely objectively "true" binary choices and then to see this for themselves by imagining clinical scenarios where this applies. If they do not come forward with their own examples of how this might be clinically relevant, the teacher might offer their own clinical example:

> It is 2 pm in the pediatric emergency room and you are a student being supervised by a resident and staff. As you review the case of an 8-month-old with a fever, you tell the resident and staff that you felt the neck was stiff on exam. You understand that if the neck is considered stiff, then a lumbar puncture (LP) will need to be done, and you would really like to observe one of these procedures. The clinical decision is a binary one – the neck is either stiff enough to require an LP or it is not. Think of what is influencing you to say that you think this infant has a stiff neck. Now compare the factors motivating you to say there is a stiff neck or not when it is 2 am in the morning instead of in the afternoon, and the same patient appears, but this time you are alone and were instructed to page the resident "if you need them," and you know that the resident is feeling overwhelmed by how busy the night has been. The mother of the child has already told you she is distrustful of antibiotics and she has no idea that you are considering the very serious diagnosis of meningitis. If an LP is required, then the consequences are to activate the resident, call the attending staff at home, have the treatment room prepared, and try to convince the parents that this test is necessary – all at 2 am. When you page the resident to discuss the case, how might these mitigating factors play into whether you think the neck is stiff or not compared to the same case that appears in the middle of the afternoon?

There are two learning points to emerge from the red exercise. First, binary choices are more complex than they initially appear. While there is nothing wrong with making binary judgments and they do need to be made, the point is to see how binary decisions are created and are not objective "truths" in and of themselves that stand on their own outside of their particular specific context. Second, knowing what to look for specifically attunes attention and results in better recognition (e.g., only when asked to specifically "look for red items" does the awareness of the large number of red items in the room become evident). A significant part of medical education is learning what to look for in patients and how to see with a clinician's eyes. The attentive neurologist, for example, may be able to make a diagnosis from observing how their patient enters the room and sits down. Recognition of the limits of any one person's capacity to pay attention and be aware also highlights how invaluable it is to seek out the thoughts and observations of others involved in patient care.

5. "Something Missed" Narrative Exercise

In this first writing exercise, the prompt is for students to think of a time when they missed something in their interaction with another person that they later realized they had not acknowledged or paid full attention to.

As this is the very first writing activity of the course, it may be helpful to explain, "Do not worry about the quality of your writing as it will not be handed in or evaluated but rather will be used only by you in the second part of the exercise to discuss in a dyad. The act of writing can help us understand an experience in a different way than simply talking about it. If you are unsure of what to write then you may find it helpful to write out the following stem as your first sentence: 'Something that I missed, or that I did not pay full attention to at the time in my interaction with another person, and only later realized that I had missed or misunderstood was the time when I ...' (and keep writing from here)."

After approximately 5–7 minutes, ask students to stop writing after they complete the sentence they are currently working on.

Students are then guided into dyads and shown how to sit almost but not quite facing each other so that they can speak quietly towards their partner's ear. We explain that we will be using this same dyad physical setup repeatedly during the rest of the course. Students are then asked to pick who will be "A" and "B" in the dyad. Students are also asked to refrain from interrupting the speaker and to consider that when one partner in a speaking-listening exercise has stopped talking and completed their story, they both will benefit from falling into silence rather than starting to talk about other non-related issues. We articulate that we are aware that in usual social situations, it can be uncomfortable and awkward to sit together in silence but that in this class sitting quietly is normal and there is no need to maintain talking. We tell students that if they continue to talk beyond the boundaries of any particular exercise, they may be taking away from the learning opportunity of their partner who might otherwise benefit from a few moments of silence. If there is an odd number of students in any particular class, one student triad may be needed in addition to the dyads. In A-B dyads the speaking-listening sequence is A-B and then B-A, while in the A-B-C triad, it is A-B and then C-A. We suggest that the teacher refrain from participating in a dyad as it is difficult to both participate in and oversee the exercise.

Once in dyads students are asked to have A read what they wrote to B. After reading out loud what they wrote, they should then feel free to expand further on the experience of having missed something. After 5 minutes the dyads are asked to stop, pause (a brief somatic anchor of attention can be used here, e.g., focused attention on the sensation of their radial pulse for 30 seconds), and then switch roles of speaker and listener (B now reads to A). When the second speaker is finished, and the dyads are mostly in silence (usually after about 5 minutes), all students are directed to return to the large group.

In the large group discussion, students are then asked, "Who would like to start off to tell their story of when they missed something?" Students are reminded, if necessary, that they are only to speak of their own story and not of their partner's. Once 3–4 students have shared their stories with the large group, some major themes are likely to have emerged. It can be highlighted that a lack of attention is more common than is often first appreciated, and that missing something that we only later realize was important or meaningful is a frequent experience.

6. Review Course Expectations and Evaluation

The course requirements in terms of what is needed to successfully pass the course are then explained to students. We point out that we have intentionally not assigned homework and that we have structured the course so that what matters most is each student's attention during class. In other words, the course requirements should be neither time intensive nor burdensome. In addition, students have access to 1–3 pages of notes for each class that were created to help them prepare for the multiple-choice questions on the end-of-course exam. The four course requirements are:

1. The course is passed when each of the three components of the course are met:

    - Student participation and engagement in each of the classes. Students are expected to engage in class exercises as best as they can. As long as they show up and are present and engaged, they will satisfy this course requirement. Students can arrange to have a separate meeting with the teacher to discuss particular issues as needed throughout the course (details on how to access teachers, such as emails, are usually offered here).
    - Passing a written essay due at the end of the course. The essay instructions will be given at Class 7 (Chap. 9) – the essay is a reflective one based on class experiences and activities.
    - Passing the multiple-choice questions on the end of pre-clerkship section exam.

2. Students need to agree to exercise what we call "double confidentiality." The teacher explains: "Regular confidentiality is when you do not discuss what other students say in class to others outside the class. In double confidentiality, you additionally agree to not bring up what a student said in class when you are both outside the class, even to them personally, unless they themselves initiate such a conversation. For example, you may feel that you want to acknowledge something that a colleague said that you thought was nice or helpful outside the classroom – but you do not know if the person who said it in class may have regretted saying it or perhaps just does not want to have it brought up outside class. Can you agree to not bring up what was said, even to the persons themselves, outside of the class?"

3. Students must arrive before the class begins. "Each class will begin exactly on time. At the time the class begins, the door will be closed and students who arrive late will not be able to join the ongoing class. This is done to ensure that late students do not disrupt classes. You may need to adjust your morning schedule to ensure that you are here early enough in order to not be late. In this course, being late means you have missed the class. Please note that there will be no exceptions once the door is closed. If when you arrive you see that the door is closed, please do not ask to be let in. Additionally, if you know you will be missing a class in advance and with faculty permission, please advise your teacher via email in advance so that your teacher is aware that you will not be attending the class."

4. No cellphones and laptops are to be used during class. "You are provided with notes for each class that will also help you study for the multiple-choice exam. Thus, there is no need for you to take notes during the class, and laptops and cellphones are to be turned off at the beginning of each class."

The most potentially contentious issue raised about the course requirements is that "being late is the same as missing a class for this course." We have found that this expectation is unique in their medical school experience to date, and many students do not like it at first! We explain that the reasons why we insist on starting on time is because entering the class late is disruptive to the small group dynamic that includes dyad work and guided awareness practices. Frequently, a student will ask, "What if there is a snowstorm or I miss my bus?" We explain that they need to leave home early enough to account for the weather and other contingencies. We suggest that they plan their day so that they may arrive early enough to not be stressed about being late – they may choose to experience what it is like to arrive 30 minutes early, for example, and do some other work or reading before class begins (note that class starts at 9:00 in the morning). We also emphasize that they will be expected to be in much earlier for most of the rest of their career when others will also be counting on them to arrive on time (e.g., for a surgeon expected in the OR or for an emergency room shift). We also emphasize that we have set a standard for being on time that we, as teachers, also need to respect and that many of us arrive an hour before class to make sure we are on time. Finally, since it is possible to pass the course with one missed class out of seven, the consequence for being late one time means that they would miss only one class, which will not impact on their ability to pass the course.

When it is time for the class to begin, the teacher closes the classroom door, and no one else may enter the class after that time. In end-of-course evaluations, students often mention how at first they did not like the no-late rule but that many of them had a change of mind once they saw for themselves how much less stressful it was to arrive early instead of just on time and to not have interruptions once the class had started. We should emphasize that we have made no exceptions to this rule, and contrary to our initial concern about feasibility, we have found it effective and helpful in creating a small group class atmosphere of respect and professionalism.

Setting course expectations and requirements to pass the course will vary between different medical school policies. We intentionally made the requirements for passing MMP to have the same criteria as any other core medical undergraduate course at McGill. That is a combination of:

- Sufficient attendance (six out of seven classes) and intra-class participation.
- Grade of at least 60% on multiple-choice exam questions.
- Passing grade of 60% on a reflective essay students hand in the week after the last class. This essay is read and graded by the MMP teacher, and personalized written feedback on each essay is given to students.

7. Cellphone Exercise in Dyads

This exercise is to be done in dyads and is the first and last time we will be using cellphones in class. For this exercise the person seated to your left is your partner. If there is an odd number, then there will also be one triad (help students arrange themselves in dyads and one triad). When you are told to start, and not until then, "A" is instructed to think of something fun or interesting that they did recently or are particularly looking forward to and be ready to tell their partner what this was. "B" is instructed to listen to "A" while at the same time catching up on their email, social media, texting, or whatever else they might want to do on their phone while "A" is telling their story. Now "A" start telling your story and "B" listen and explore your phone at the same time.

After 3–5 minutes ask students to stop. Do not debrief. Then have them switch roles and begin again for 3–5 minutes. A large group debrief then begins by asking how it was to be the person who was telling their story, "What was it like to be talking to someone who was on their phone? What did you notice?" Then ask how it felt to be the person on the phone while the other person was telling their story. What did they notice?

This exercise has students experience what it feels like to listen while simultaneously paying partial attention to other stimuli on their cellphone and then secondly to experience telling an interesting story to a listener whose attention is being pulled in different directions. In the structured debrief, when asked what they noticed as the listener, typical responses range from, "It was easy." to "It was very difficult and uncomfortable." Most students state that they find scanning their phone while someone is talking to them to be an unpleasant and less than satisfying experience. Others state that they find it quite normal and they are comfortable with it. When asked to reflect on what it was like to be the storyteller, many students describe feeling a need to increase the drama of their story in order to try to compete for attention as it felt that the listener was finding more interesting things to look at on their phone rather than paying full attention to their story. Other students share that they gave up telling their story when they felt that they were not being heard. At the conclusion of this exercise, the negative effects of being distracted are generally self-evident, and it is an easy segue for the teacher to then state that in the future cellphones will be turned off at the start of each class.

The cellphone exercise is a hands-on way for students to examine their experience of paying intermittent or partial instead of full attention, and it fits in well in this introductory class on the limits of attentional capacity. The class discussion often leads to questions of the validity of the "myth of multitasking" versus rapid switching of attention between multiple tasks idea. In Class 5 (Chap. 7) on building resilience, they will experience a dyad exercise that will have them listen and speak with finely tuned attention in order for them to again experience for themselves the different aspects of speaking and listening with partial versus full attention. We find that these speaking and listening experiences with shifting levels of attention are one way to have students learn "listening skills," which while lauded as being of high importance for the good clinician, are rarely explicitly taught.

8. Brief GAP

The teacher guides a 2–3-minute GAP focused on the sensation of the breath. At the end of this GAP, there is no debrief. The teacher might signal the end of the class by saying, "I wish you a good day and will see you next week."

See Table 3.1, teaching template for Class 1.

Table 3.1 Teaching template. Class 1: Attention and Awareness

Core concepts	Materials	Time,
Course intentions	Change blindness video	Minutes
Attentional capacity	Paper, pens, markers	
Mindfulness and multitasking		

Note: allow latecomers and cellphones only for this first class

1. Introducing the MMP class
"Say your name and what it means to you."
"What is this course about?" (learning skills on how to be a better MD)
Optional additional questions:
    "Why is MMP offered at this time in the curriculum?" (before clerkship = just right)
    "In what possible clinical scenarios might your capacity to pay attention be important?"
	15

2. Guided awareness practice Seated body scan and breath meditation Debrief: "What did you notice?"	10
3. Change blindness video (https://www.youtube.com/watch?v=1nL5ulsWMYc) "What are possible clinical correlates to this phenomenon?" (e.g., a patient gradually becoming cyanosed while you are taking their history)	10
4. Four minutes of red exercise In silence, encourage standing up and walking around Large group: 3 students with longest lists write them on whiteboard Share and compare "Were you surprised by how much red there was?" (impact of primed looking) "How did you decide what was red enough to list?" Thresholds and decision-making: make clinical connection to so-called binary choices (e.g., LP for "stiff neck") and impact of contextual influences	15

5. "Something missed" narrative exercise
"Think of a time when you missed something in an interaction you had with another person. It could be what was said to you that you only later realized you had missed or misinterpreted or not fully heard. What you missed may have come out of a clinical or a personal interaction."
    Offer sentence-starting stem
    Ensure all are writing – give 5–7 min
    Dyads share writing: A-B and then B-A (5 min each)
    Large group: students share examples
    Make connection to clinical settings; medical errors when we ignore in the moment what later appears obvious
	20

6. Review course expectations and evaluation (1) Attendance and participation, essay, final exam (2) Explain double confidentiality (3) Classes start exactly on time; door closed = missed class (4) Cellphones off; no laptops (notes provided)	10
7. Cellphone exercise in dyads (5 min each) Debrief listener and multitasker Point out that being listened to is not just "nice" but is a physician's responsibility Cellphones to be turned off in future classes	15
8. Brief GAP (2–3 min) No debrief "I wish you a good day and will see you next week."	5

Reference

1. Simons DJ, Franconeri SL, Reimer RL. Gradual change test 2000. https://youtu. be/1nL5ulsWMYc. Accessed 21 August 2018.

Chapter 4
Class 2: Congruent Communication

Tom A. Hutchinson

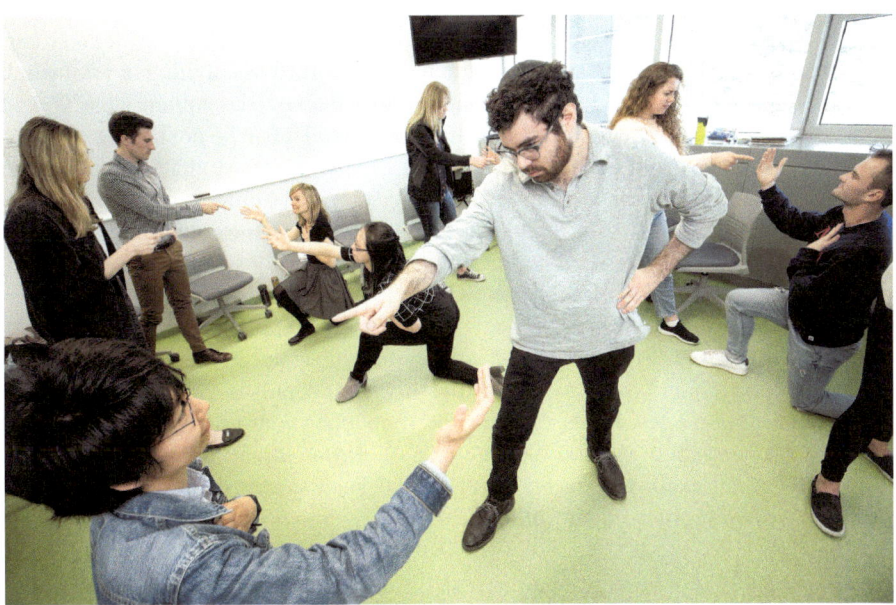

Fig. 4.1 Multiple student pairs in blaming and placating stances

Overview

In this class we are moving students from primarily external awareness as typified by the noticing red and other exercises in the first class to internal awareness and demonstrating how it impacts relationships with other people including patients using the Satir communication stances (Fig. 4.1). This can be a difficult step for some students to take and

© Springer Nature Switzerland AG 2020
S. Liben, T. A. Hutchinson, *MD Aware*,
https://doi.org/10.1007/978-3-030-22430-1_4

is occurring at an early stage in the course before the teacher has a sense of each individual student. The teacher probably does not yet know all of their names. We have found that it is particularly important to deliberately slow ourselves down and become conscious of our own internal processes in this important second class in the course. The tendency when we become anxious, particularly if we suppress the anxiety, is to speed up and teach this material superficially. Your anxiety may be triggered particularly when you repeat from the first class the question "What is the purpose of this course?" and receive very little in the way of a response. If this happens, wait longer than is completely comfortable, and in our experience, there is always at least one response. Whatever response you get, treat it very positively and very seriously, which will likely encourage other students to respond. But even if you have very little response from students at this point, do not be alarmed. Remind yourself that what you are seeing is not likely due to lack of interest but to anxiety on the part of the students.

The second time in this class when it is important to slow down and keep your focus is when you have students act out some of the Satir communication stances in step 4 (see Section "4 Satir Stances"). What Satir would call "sculpting" feels strange and uncomfortable to some students, which may manifest as laughing or joking, taking a bathroom break, or looking unhappy or disinterested. Explain what you are doing and beware of paying too much attention to students who are having difficulty with the process in some way. Be clear about what you want students to do and proceed at a deliberate pace. Beware of speeding up in an attempt to retain students' attention. We will return to communication stances later in the course, and this initial experience of the stances is an important building block for what comes later.

A final piece of advice in teaching Class 2. Because this is early in the process and students are still getting to know you and the course, do not be surprised if they seem a little cautious. Beware of concluding that this is not a good or open group of students. Surprisingly, we have found that this is especially a danger after you have taught the course a few times. It is easy to remember your previous groups of students as they were at the end of the course and to compare them with the group before you. Of course, you may well make such comparisons and have such thoughts, but don't take them too seriously.

1. One Word that Describes the Purpose of this Course

"What is the purpose of this course?" We begin the class by asking students a question that is similar to the one we asked in the first class. The answers will be fairly similar to the first class with more seriousness in their responses. They have usually by this stage given up the illusion that the course is primarily about relaxation. They will respond with words such as mindfulness, paying attention, and awareness. We will pick up on responses such as paying attention or awareness to ask a follow-up question, "Awareness of what?" Students will give examples from the last class but may not mention awareness of themselves. Whether or not this comes up, we raise it as the main purpose of this class.

Starting with a question that is similar to the question posed in the first class does two things. First, it reinforces that we are asking the students to think and reflect. Although there are didactic elements in this course, our primary teaching method is to listen to the students and use what they say to move the class forward. To facilitate this process and to encourage individual students to speak, we almost never reject or disagree with what a student says. Instead we attempt to find something helpful in whatever is said. Second, the benefit of asking a similar question is that it creates surprise ("I thought we already answered that question"). The element of surprise is an important part of our teaching method that helps keep students awake and alert. The surprise in the response to this question is that there is more to awareness than external awareness. Medical students' awareness tends to be turned outwards, and they often have more difficulty focusing on their own body sensations and emotions. We emphasize that this course is not just about external awareness and exploration but internal exploration that is very important for their development as physicians. This discussion leads easily into the first guided awareness in this class, where they turn their attention internally.

2. Guided Awareness Practice

We lead this short guided awareness practice (GAP) by asking students to begin noticing their bodies sitting in the chair and any body sensations that they have. We start with the sensations in their toes, to feet, to lower legs, and progressively on up to their abdomens. We move from there to breath awareness. The breath is the ongoing focus, but we ask students to notice sensations, thoughts, or emotions that may come and go as they focus on their breath.

3. Reacting Versus Responding

We explain briefly the difference between reacting (an unconscious and unchosen way that we automatically find ourselves behaving or being when an event or interaction with another person occurs) and responding (a conscious and deliberately chosen response to an event or interaction). We draw a simple diagram on the board as shown in Fig. 4.2. We follow this by an example from our own lives of a recent reaction. This is not hard to find as we are all reacting, at least internally, most of the time in our day-to-day lives. Students will normally assume that the purpose of the class is to prevent or suppress reactions. We emphasize that this is not the case.

We suggest a different approach: pause, notice our reaction, and then, without suppression, make a choice about how to proceed. An example from our own lives can be very helpful. A typical example would be as follows: "I was on the phone to

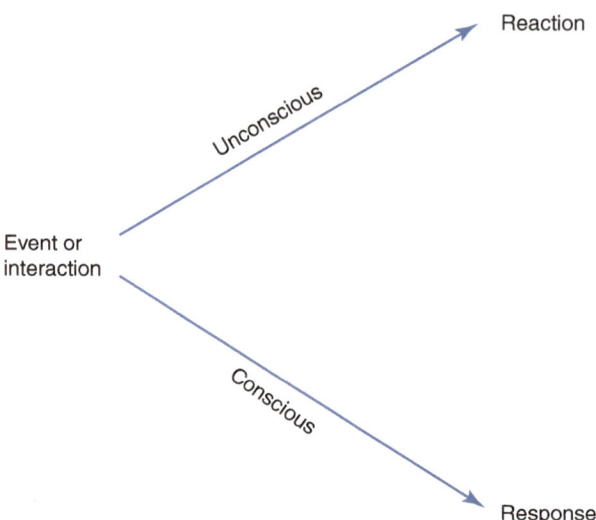

Fig. 4.2 Reaction versus response

a travel agent who was trying to help me plan an itinerary for a trip. She was talking a lot, often to herself, pointing out difficulties, using codes for flights that I did not understand. I could feel myself becoming tense and frustrated. Rather than acting on my reaction or simply suppressing it as I continued to listen, I paused, registered my reaction and thought about a reasonable response. I stopped my travel agent for a moment with gentleness and told her that I believed she was clear on what my main requirements were. Why didn't I give her some time to work on a few alternatives and get back to me when she was ready." This did not make me wrong (for getting frustrated) or her wrong (for the messy process of trying to find a solution) and was a better use of both our time – a helpful response versus a potentially harmful reaction.

We then divide the class into pairs and ask them to share with each other an experience where they reacted to a person or event. We ask them to pick a recent example; it may not be clinical but should be a relatively powerful example of an unchosen reaction. We then debrief some of these reactions in the large group. Mostly we are listening to what individual students report, but we often have follow-up questions to clarify what happened and to show interest, which must be real, not feigned. After four or five such reports, which will probably be quite different and from different contexts, we make the observation that the way of reacting with which they are most familiar is with anger. If it has not already come up, we ask for reactions that did not involve overt anger. If an example is shared, we discuss it. If not, we ask how many students have found themselves automatically saying "yes" when they meant "no." Many students will normally confirm that they have done this. We point out that this is another automatic way of reacting. In fact, there are a number of automatic ways of reacting that we will now describe.

4. Satir Stances

Since we give the students a brief background on Virginia Satir, a family therapist who identified different automatic stances that people take when interacting with another person we suggest that anyone teaching this course should familiarize themselves with the work of Virginia Satir. Although the concepts that we teach based on Satir's work are relatively simple, one needs to have a sense of Satir's overall philosophy and way of viewing people to impart the full impact of this material. One good way to start to get a sense for this is to read her book *The New Peoplemaking* or at a minimum read Chaps. 7 and 8 in that book [1].

However, to teach this material effectively, the teacher needs more than cognitive understanding. The situation is analogous to the teaching of mindfulness, which can only be effectively taught, we believe, by someone who has participated in formal mindfulness training. For the teaching of Satir's communication stances and congruence, a similar experiential background is important. For one of the coauthors (TAH), this consisted of participation in a 4-day workshop with Virginia Satir in the 1980s and subsequent participation in workshops and courses led by some of Virginia's colleagues and coworkers in Ottawa (Janet Seely) and Vancouver (John Banmen). There are also multiple and ongoing opportunities for new and future Mindful Medical Practice (MMP) teachers to join Satir-based training workshops available by searching the World Wide Web. In our group at McGill, the experiential aspect of Satir's teaching has been disseminated through workshops and courses in which mindfulness and congruence have been taught experientially to faculty including those who subsequently became MMP course instructors. We believe that such experiential learning is essential to teach this material effectively.

A second element is also required. Just as with mindfulness, taking a course is insufficient. Further and continued practice is required. This means attempting to notice one's own stances in day-to-day life and making choices that foster better relationships, including bringing congruence into our everyday and intimate relationships. Only in this way can we appreciate both the difficulty of being congruent and the powerful benefits that it can bring to our relationships. We believe that continued experiential exploration is essential to bring life and authenticity to the teaching of the Satir material.

We begin this exercise by offering students a very brief background on the work of Virginia Satir, explaining that she was a family therapist who identified different automatic stances that people take in interacting with another person. We draw on the board a circle divided into three parts: self, other, and context, as shown in Fig. 4.3. We point out that it would seem fairly straightforward to stay in contact with these three elements (congruence) – ourselves as a person, the other person as a person, and the context – but in fact to be congruent is much more difficult than it appears. Particularly under stress, we drop out one or more of the three elements to the detriment of the interaction and the relationship. We then draw on the board the four communication stances as shown in Fig. 4.4. In the placating stance, we leave out ourselves as a per-

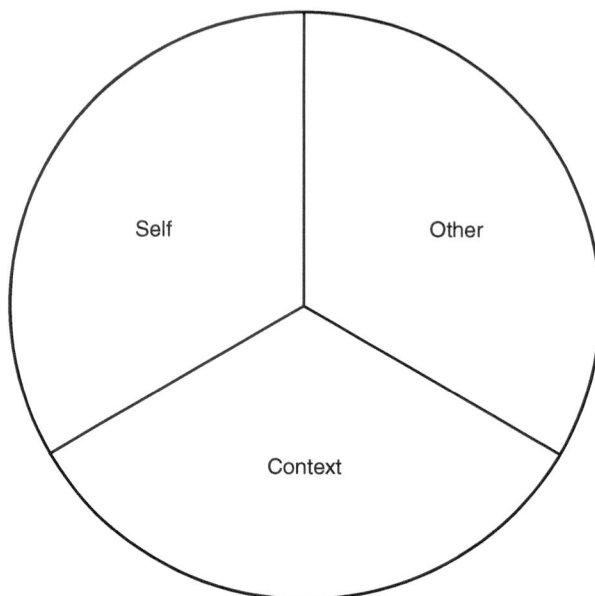

Fig. 4.3 Present to the three elements in an interaction – congruent

son. We point out that this is the starting point for many medical students who wish to do their best for the patient. However, it is difficult to continue to behave in this way over a period of time and is often not what patients want. They want to experience us as a person.

Sometimes after a period of placating in our lives, we may become sufficiently unhappy with this self-suppression that we move to a contrasting stance – the blaming stance. Now we want the other person to meet our expectations. In medicine this may manifest as labelling the patient or family as dysfunctional, difficult, or non-compliant. This may be true, but it may also mean we are automatically adopting a blaming stance.

We now move to the super-reasonable stance in which we leave out ourselves as a person and the other person as a person. We point out that in medicine there is sometimes a desire to avoid emotion and thus effectively to avoid being present to ourselves and the patient as a person. We ask the students whether they have seen this in a clinical context. Almost always students are very familiar with this stance in clinical medicine. If not, we can give our own favorite example. One example is a neurologist discussing in the presence of the patient the possible location of the lesion in a patient with a stroke with his or her residents. This ignores the humanity of the patient but also of the physician. We point out that although this stance appears to solve a problem (avoid the interference of emotions), it can be extremely upsetting when a person is confronting a frightening and emotionally powerful diagnosis or medical problem.

We then come to the final stance, the distracting stance, in which we lose touch with everything: ourselves as a person; the other person as a person; and the context. We point out that this is not as rare as we might hope in clinical practice. There are various ways

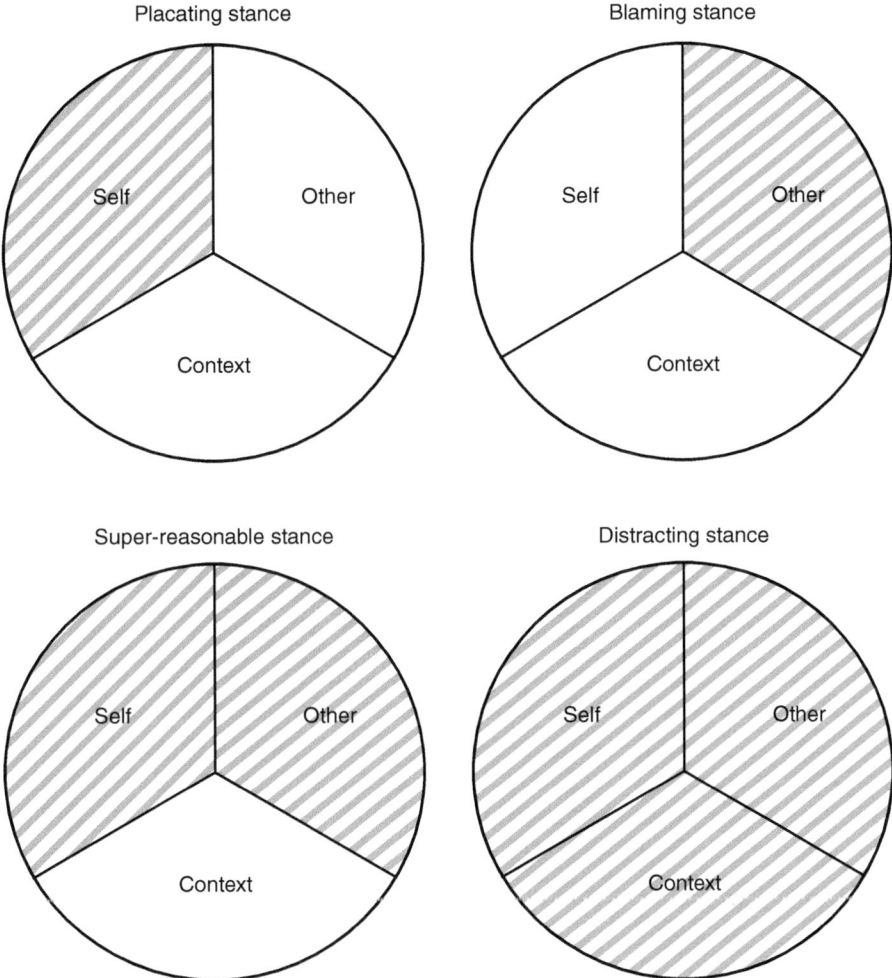

Fig. 4.4 Communication stances

this manifests, such as extreme multitasking, particularly with electronic media, and at times completely inappropriate jokes. We ask students if they have seen this, and normally they will easily come up with examples. If not, we can supply a favorite one of our own. We point out that one way of looking at these stances is that we are progressively leaving out more of the interaction: ourselves as a person, the other person as a person, both ourselves and the other person as persons, and both people in the interaction as persons plus the context. We clarify that the ideal interaction is one in which we stay present to all three elements – what Virginia Satir would call "congruence."

We find that the stances are intuitively easy for students to relate to and easy for them to recognize in their clinical and other life experience. They can easily see that leaving out one or more elements in an interaction, although intended to make things easier, usually makes things worse. However, we may make a point here, or later, that adopting a stance is not always bad. Stances have their uses, and our objective is to be able to pause, notice what is being left out, and make a choice about how to proceed.

Sometimes students point out that there are possible combinations of self, other, and context that are not covered by the stances. These involve leaving out the context while being present to other elements such as self only, other only, and both self and other. Some people have suggested that being present to self and other but losing touch with the context describes being in love. We acknowledge these other possibilities if they are raised by the students but do not pursue a long conversation about them. We do not want to turn this into an abstract intellectual exercise. We wish to teach them the basic stances and particularly their subjective experience of these stances, which leads naturally to the next part of this section.

We point out that the stances come with a physical posture that helps give an experience of the particular reactive stance. The physical postures associated with each stance are given in Fig. 4.5. We first act out each of the first three stances ourselves: placating is down on the right knee, right hand over the heart, left hand reaching up to someone else, and apologizing; blaming is one hand on the hip with the other hand pointing at another person and being overtly angry; super-reasonable or computer brain is looking above the person and thinking interesting analytical thoughts.

We now break the group into pairs and distribute the pairs throughout the room. Students pick an A and a B. Student A takes the placating stance and student B the blaming stance. Without words they hold the stance in silence for 1 minute noticing their body sensations and emotions. We then reverse A and B with A now blaming and B placating. Again, they hold the stances in silence for 1 minute. We now ask A to change from blaming to super-reasonable, which means looking above the person without making eye contact. Again, they hold their stance for 1 minute in silence. We ask the students who are in the placating stance if they preferred it when the other person was blaming or super-reasonable. Most students prefer to be blamed than treated as a nonperson in the super-reasonable stance, an important insight for relating to patients.

Getting the students to adopt the physical stances is fun, insightful, and potentially disruptive. It is important to give very clear and firm instructions, to emphasize silence and noticing body sensations and emotions as they hold the stances, and to immediately intervene if students are laughing and joking. You might make the point that if they notice themselves laughing, they are probably feeling uncomfortable and reacting by adopting the distracting stance, which is not called for in this exercise. We have found that it is most effective to do this exercise with pairs of students distributed throughout the room. If there is an uneven number of students, we suggest that either the instructor complete a pair, while still leading the group (this takes some skill), or have one group of three students with the person observing changing as you go through the different combinations of stances.

We have students again sit in a circle and report on what they noticed. Acting out the stances can be very insightful and can also make some students uncomfortable; both of these effects may come up in the large group discussion. Some students will feel very familiar with the placating stance. We stress that this is not bad. They are learning something about themselves. Some students may be very uncomfortable

Placating   Blaming

Super-reasonable   Distracting

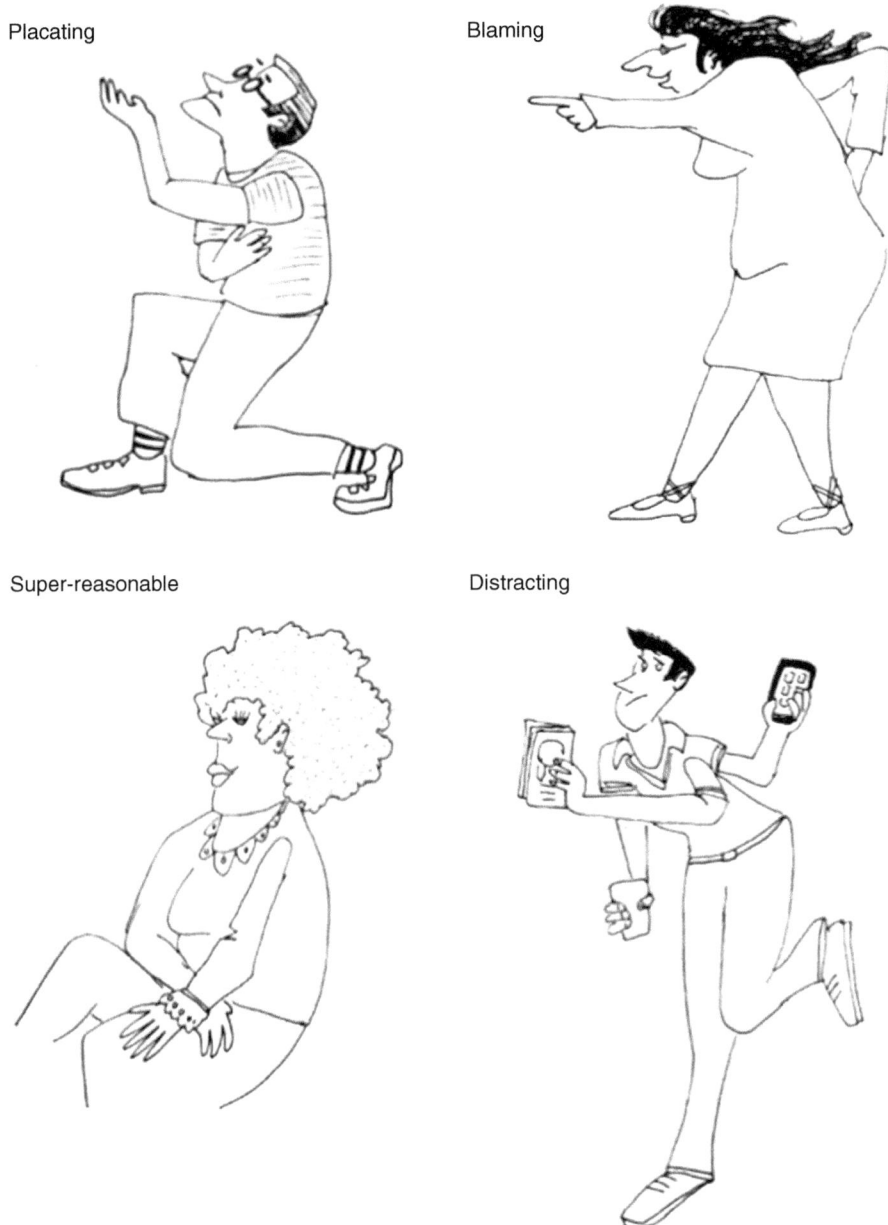

Fig. 4.5 Communication stances: physical postures. (Adapted by Chris Tucker from Satir [1])

taking up the blaming stance. We have even had participants virtually incapable of acting out this stance. It is important not to go with the conclusion that the blaming stance is always bad. All the stances have a function, and the blaming stance may be effective with a confused or panicking person who needs very clear direction or as a step towards congruence in someone who habitually placates. We point out that the aim is to familiarize ourselves with all the stances so that we may recognize when we are in a stance, and notice which stances seem familiar and comfortable (often our own frequently used stance or stances), and notice which stances seem unfamiliar and uncomfortable (an opportunity to explore possible areas of growth for us). The most important objective is to notice when we are in a stance and then to decide if our response will be a continuation of that stance or to add the missing part to produce congruence. We make the point that on balance congruence probably works best in most interactions – both in the immediate interaction and as a contribution to the long-term relationship.

5. Mindfulness and Congruence

We ask students how mindfulness relates to these stances and to congruence. Students easily pick up that the purpose is to pause for self-awareness so that they can make a decision whether to stay in a reactive stance or add in the missing part.

In introducing this guided meditation, we make the analogy between distraction in meditation and reaction. We ask students to focus on the sensations of the body sitting in a chair and to notice distractions as reactions about which they can consciously make a choice: either go with the thought or other distraction or return to focus on body sensation. Looked at this way, every distraction during guided awareness can be viewed as a mini-reaction that students first notice before deciding whether to return to focus on the body sensations. We emphasize that they are exercising a pause muscle that will be useful not just in meditation but in staying self-aware when they interact with patients and others in a clinical context.

This is followed by a discussion between pairs of students. We change the dyad configurations at this point because students will often have paired up with friends and we want students to have one-on-one experience with as many other students in the group as possible. The changing configuration is particularly important when we notice two students who appear not to be sufficiently involved in the class and who may be supporting each other in their nonengagement. Identifying an A and a B, we give each of them 2 minutes to reflect on their experience in the guided awareness. We then debrief in the large group what came up in the GAP and how what they learned today may be relevant to clinical practice. This should be a fairly brief discussion (5 minutes). Do not be concerned if this turns out to be a shorter class (scheduled for 1 hour and 45 minutes but may be shorter by 10 or 15 minutes). The main impact of this class comes from acting out the communication stances, and we do not wish to reduce this effect by a prolonged final discussion.

See Table 4.1, Teaching template for Class 2.

Table 4.1 Teaching template. Class 2: Congruent Communication

Core concepts	Materials	Time
Reacting versus responding Communication stances Congruence	Whiteboard markers Self-confidence!	Minutes
1. One word that describes the purpose of this course Highlight that we are learning to work with attention and awareness as clinically essential during patient encounters Awareness of self in particular in this class		10
2. Guided awareness practice Guided body scan from feet to abdomen finishing with attention to the breath		10
3. Reacting versus responding Draw on whiteboard and offer personal example "Recall a recent episode where you <u>reacted</u> (versus responded) to another person and what that person said or did." AB dyads (silent listener): 2 min. each A-B and B-A		15
Have students relate some of these experiences in the larger group If what emerges is that anger or frustration are the most commonly recognized reactions, then ask: "What are other ways of reacting besides anger?" (One answer is placating – automatically saying "yes" when they mean "no")		10

4. Satir stances
Background to Satir's work on communication stances
Describe framework of self, other, and context
Make a simple drawing on the whiteboard of placating, blaming, super-reasonable, and distracting
"How have you noticed these stances in clinical situations?"
Demonstrate the physical posture of each stance to students
Students then act out stances in dyads:
    A: blaming, B: placating. Reverse. "In what way do they feel different?"
    A: placating, B: change from blaming to super-reasonable. Ask A (placating) "Who do you prefer to be with, the blamer or the super-reasonable person?"
    Most placaters prefer to be paired with a blamer than a super-reasonable person.
		30

"What did you notice in doing this exercise?" Discuss the aim: Once consciously aware of a stance, there is a choice: either stay in the stance or replace the missing awareness to produce congruence		10
5. Mindfulness and congruence "How does mindfulness fit into the process of stances and congruence?" Make analogy of distraction in meditation and reaction GAP – exercising the "pause" muscle Final dyad discussion with pairs changed		20

Reference

1. Satir V. The new peoplemaking. Mountain View: Science and Behavior Books; 1988.

Chapter 5
Class 3: Awareness and Decision-Making

Stephen Liben

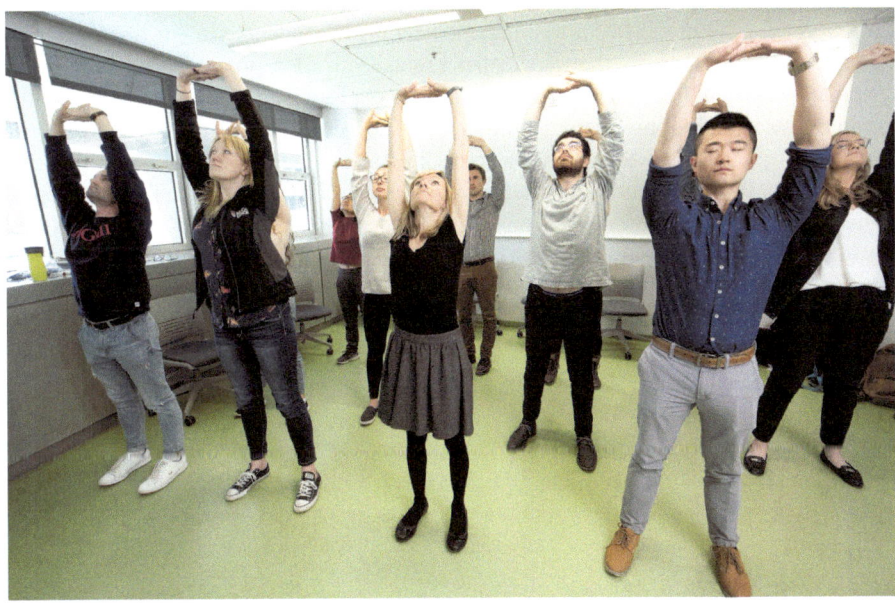

Fig. 5.1 Students with arms raised in guided mindful movement

Overview

This third class, Awareness and Decision-Making, makes a connection between awareness of body sensations practiced in Classes 1 and 2 (Chaps. 3 and 4) using body scans
and breath awareness to the process of clinical decision-making (Fig. 5.1). To our
knowledge, standard medical education rarely explores the role of the clinician's own

© Springer Nature Switzerland AG 2020
S. Liben, T. A. Hutchinson, *MD Aware*,
https://doi.org/10.1007/978-3-030-22430-1_5

moment-to-moment body sensations in both consciously and unconsciously influencing behavior and decision-making. Standard medical education instead tends to focus on what students think about disease processes that are occurring in their patients' bodies. The question usually asked of students in clinical encounters is "What do you think is going on with the patient?" rather than "What body sensations are you aware of as you interact with this patient?" The *embodied* physician is aware not only of the contents of their thoughts but also of their interoceptive (internal sensations, such as sensing one's own rapid heartbeat) and exteroceptive (external sensations, such as noticing cyanosis in a patient) perceptions. An underexplored area in medical education is how interoceptive and exteroceptive sensory awareness might be helpful in clinician-patient communication, medical decision-making, and avoiding medical errors. This class asks, "What is the role of awareness of internal and external body sensations in medical decision-making?" What colloquially is referred to as "gut instinct" speaks to the commonality of the experience of suspecting when something is wrong "because it just feels wrong," even when the cognitive reason cannot be easily articulated. By examining a video reenactment of a real-life medical error, students see for themselves the connected web of errors that led to the brain death of a previously healthy young woman. The idea that we encourage students to explore is the danger of ignoring their own physical sensations when making medical decisions. This is not to say that sensations and gut instincts are always correct, but rather that *sensations are a source of information* that can be assessed once brought to conscious awareness. With the appearance in consciousness of a sensation (e.g., "My hands are very sweaty"), the next step is to examine more closely what that could mean (e.g., "I wonder if I am nervous about something that I was not even fully aware of"). The mindfully aware, embodied clinician is monitoring thoughts, emotions, and physical sensations as sources of information that may or not be helpful or correct on further examination. Without the three different aspects of experience held in awareness – thoughts, emotional states, and physical sensations (see Triangle of Attention, Chap. 7, Class 5) – there is a loss of potentially useful information to help guide clinical decision-making. By paying mindful attention to their own physical sensations, we hope that students will be less error-prone and will not have the experience commonly expressed by clinical colleagues after a mistake is made: "I just knew it in my gut, but I ignored the warning signs."

1. Guided Awareness Practice

The class begins with a 10-minute guided awareness practice (GAP) that focuses on bringing attention repeatedly back to the felt sensation of the breath (as air movements felt at the nostrils or as the abdomen rises and falls with each breath). At the conclusion of the exercise, the teacher explains the difference between *formal* and *informal* awareness practices.

(a) *Formal awareness practice*, or formal meditation, occurs in a controlled setting for a specific predetermined period of time such as practiced together at the beginning of each class. Formal practice is the cultivation of the ability to pay attention and increase awareness through scheduled, concentrated practice exercises while sustaining attention on an attentional "anchor" or focus. Attentional anchors are most often a physical sensation felt or sensed in the present moment (the present being the only time that such sensations can be perceived, we cannot feel the pain of tomorrow's toothache before it arises). A commonly used physical sensation, or attentional "anchor," is the sensation of the breath as air moves past the lips or under the nose or as the abdomen rises and falls with each inspiration and expiration. Physical sensations such as the breath are uniquely helpful as they are always arising and fading away within awareness (showing their impermanence), and unlike thoughts that carry the mind away from the present moment towards events in the past or future, physical sensations happen only now and are always accessible. Formal practices include sitting, standing, lying down, or walking meditations; body scans; and mindful movement (yoga).

(b) *Informal awareness practices* are brief periods of intentionally bringing attention to specific felt sensations in the moment as experienced in activities of daily living (e.g., the sensation of water running between your fingers as you wash your hands before examining a patient). This attentional focus is contrasted with the usual default mode of the mind that is "lost in thought." An example of being lost in thought would be when a movie is being watched and the watcher forgets they are in a theater with other people as they become immersed in the movie's storyline. When the movie ends, and the lights go back on, there is often a moment of remembering context and place that was willfully suspended during the movie, experienced as "Oh right, I am in a movie theatre." Such periods of "being lost in thought" may make up much of conscious experience within a regular day, and informal practices are a "stepping outside" of the lost mode of mind that is immersed in the *content* of thoughts, in order to willfully bring awareness to the thinking process itself. In other words, unlike focused attention on *what* thoughts are (the default mode that concentrates on contents of a thought) being mindful is an awareness *that* thoughts are occurring. An example of an informal practice would be just before entering the room of a patient when attention can be purposively brought to the felt sensation of the doorknob (perceived as cold or warm or smooth) as felt on the hand, pausing to note the sensation and the presence of thoughts and the emotional state in the moment, and then proceeding to enter the room (these are components of the "STOP" exercise described further in Chap. 7, Class 5). There are many other opportunities for such informal practices through the day, and at first glance it may appear that this is all that is needed to be more "mindful."

The question may be asked, why not just tell oneself to practice informally and avoid having to set time aside for formal practice at all? While it is reasonable to imagine that all that is needed to be mindful during the day is to do more informal practices, it can be pointed out that without some formal practice, it is unlikely that the intention to practice informally will actually occur with any regularity. Formal practices serve as a support and catalyst to increase the capacity for informal awareness practice. The goal of both formal and informal practice is to increase the capacity for moment-to-moment mindful awareness within any activity.

2. Check In

Check in with students by asking, "Has anything come up in relation to class last week, or so far in the course, that you would like to ask or talk about?" This offers the opportunity for students to express doubts and to clarify misconceptions. We find that students only occasionally bring up specific questions, but when they do, they are often questions or issues that others in the class are also experiencing but may not be comfortable asking about or sharing with the group. At this point in the course, common misconceptions often remain such as that awareness exercises are "about relaxing" (versus the true goal of being aware of any state of being rather than aiming for any particular or relaxed state) or that the course is about self-care (the main focus is rather on helping students develop specific clinical skills). Other misconceptions of the awareness practices themselves may also come up such as that it is easy to have the mind focused steadily on the breath for 10 minutes. The idea that "I am having no thoughts and meditation is easy" is a common experience for first time meditators who may not be aware that their mind is drifting into thought during a 10-minute meditation. It may take several sessions for enough awareness to develop to even be aware that attentional focus on the breath is inevitably repeatedly being lost into thoughts and then needs to be redirected back to the sensation of the breath. It can be pointed out that students who have questions or concerns are welcome to reach the teacher after class and that separate face-to-face meetings may also be arranged.

3. Awareness and Medical Errors

Factors that result in medical errors are complex and multifactorial and relate to the interaction of systems (e.g., electronic prescribing) with the limitations of human decision-making (e.g., the known increase in prescription medication error rate when the clinician is distracted). While the science of medical errors is still in evolution and improvements in systems should help to reduce the current very high incidence of medical errors [1], the role of the individual's capacity to be as aware as possible of what is happening in the moment remains essential and within everyone's own personal locus of control. Students may be asked, "How common are medical errors?" as an introduction to the theme of this class. Students typically know that medical errors are a common cause of morbidity and mortality but may not be aware of just how frequently they rank in the top 3–5 causes of death in the USA.

Our understanding of how and which mental and physical bodily processes are involved when a decision is being made continues to evolve. There are somatic markers, such as palm sweating measured in the galvanic skin response (GSR; sweat gland output that correlates with emotional arousal), that occur in the absence of conscious awareness.

The Iowa gambling task is then explained by the teacher as an example of how an *unconscious* physical sensation, in this case a GSR indicating palm sweating that

correlates with anxiety, increased before a "bad decision" came to *conscious* awareness in the controlled experiment [2]. We explain to students that subjects were
presented with four decks of cards (we draw four decks of cards onto the whiteboard
to help illustrate the experiment and how subjects in the experiment made decisions) and told that each deck held cards that would either reward or penalize them
with varying amounts of money. The goal was to win as much money as possible,
and they were able to choose cards as they wished from each of the four decks. What
they did not know is that the four decks differed from each other in that two of the
four decks were "better" in terms giving steady positive payouts, while the other
two decks had big losses or much smaller gains. Most subjects started off by sam-
pling cards from each of the four decks, and after about 50 selections, subjects were
able to state which were the "better paying" two decks. However, what was surprising was that subjects' GSR demonstrated a stress reaction when their hands were
hovering above the two "bad decks" *after only ten cards*, long before they were
consciously aware that specific decks were bad choices (an awareness that only
become conscious after 40–50 cards). This phenomenon suggests that there is information present (good versus bad card choices) that is manifested in physical
responses (sweating) significantly *before* (about 30 card choices before) such
knowledge is available to conscious perception.

The influence on decision-making of bringing physical sensations to conscious
awareness has been explored in the somatic marker hypothesis [3]. Additionally,
neuroscientific data showing a relationship between conscious awareness of one's
own physical sensations such as breathing and heartbeat and the capacity to attune
to the somatic and affective states of others raises the possibility of a positive correlation between interoceptive awareness and empathy [4, 5]. Intentionally bringing
focused attention to physical sensations has traditionally been used in contemplative Buddhist practices to allow a specific type of awareness (mindfulness) to
emerge in seeing thoughts as thoughts, sensations as sensations, and emotions as
emotions. Mindful awareness that thoughts, sensations, and emotions are a form of
information, in and of themselves neither necessarily true nor false, helps develop
the capacity to discern and respond rather than react as if each thought, sensation,
and emotion were correct. In an evolving medical situation where there is a felt
sense (a "gut reaction") from the clinician that something is wrong, the mindfully
aware clinician would pause briefly to better discern what else may be going on in
the moment (by widening attention) and only then decide what and if any further
action might be helpful.

4. Narrative Exercise

This is a narrative exercise where students are each asked to write out the description of an experience based on the following prompt: "Think of a time when you
made an assumption, or jumped to a conclusion, and then later found out it was a
mistake. For example, you may have felt a need to apologize to someone; or perhaps
you realized later that you should have said something or spoken up when you had
chosen to be silent."

Students are then given about 6 minutes to write out their experience on their own. Once the 6 minutes are complete, we then pair students into dyads and have them identify who will be "A" and who will be "B." We ask student A to share exactly what they wrote with student B for 3 minutes, while B remains silent. We instruct A that once they have read what they wrote to B, they can then add their own commentary or additional thoughts to tell B. We advise B to be careful not comment on A's story or to tell their own story, but rather to only ask questions that would help A better understand what their experience was like *for them*. In other words, B asks A questions about their story not because of B's curiosity, but rather with the intention to help A better understand what their story may have been about on deeper levels and why they might have chosen it. Once the 3 minutes are complete, the teacher then creates a mindful pause by directing students to briefly and purposely direct their attention to the physical sensation of their feet on the floor. After the pause, we ask student B to read what they wrote to A as described above, for an additional 3 minutes.

A large group debrief follows where students are encouraged to share their experience in the dyad. Note that, as always, students are directed to not share what their partner in a dyad said or wrote. After a few stories have been shared with the large group, then students are asked, "How do assumptions/biases/jumping to conclusions with incomplete data (such as you may have noticed in the red exercise from last class) influence how you make decisions?"

The point of this narrative exercise is to bring out the phenomenon that jumping to a conclusion that is based on very little information, but much interpretation, is often the root cause of misunderstandings. The distance from a brief observation (e.g., someone driving very slowly in front of you when you are in a hurry) to a narrowed selected interpretation and then assumption and conclusion (e.g., that slow driver must be either oblivious to others or looking at his phone) to an action (e.g., honking your car horn at them to hurry up) often occurs within seconds and often leads to unhelpful conclusions and actions. Such rapid escalation from an observation to an action based on a chain of assumptions is often fraught with error and regret. Formal awareness practices as practiced in each class are intended to provide students with a "mindful pause button" where, in the moment just after an observation, they bring attention to what they are thinking, feeling, and sensing in their body. This mindful pause allows for questioning of assumptions and beliefs that may or may not be true or helpful upon further examination. Pausing to become aware of assumptions is not meant to impede action but rather to have actions based on a better understanding of the range of explanations underlying observations.

5. Medical Error Video

The 14-minute medical error video "Just a Routine Operation" [6] is a documentary narrated by Martin Bromiley, an airplane captain, whose wife Elaine died unexpectedly during what should have been a routine operation. A subsequent inquest established that her death was the direct result of both human factors and systemic failures in the healthcare system. The video that we show uninterrupted to students includes a reenactment of the operation. The documentary is emotionally powerful both because of the high quality of the reenactment and also because of the heartfelt narration by the man who lost his wife due to the types of system-communication errors he was specifically trained to avoid in his own career as an airline pilot.

Just before the video, we tell students that in the discussion to follow, we will ask them to reflect on the three components of conscious experience of which they can be aware from moment to moment. The components of experience we ask them to pay particular attention to as they view the video are their thoughts, emotions, and physical sensations, which make up the Triangle of Attention (Chap. 7, Class 5).

Debriefing the Video with the Large Group

Once the video is complete, we ask the large group of students to reflect back on whether they remembered to pay attention to the three separate components of their experience and, if some forgot to do so, to notice how easy it is, in the moment and despite their intention to pay attention, to lose the ability to discern between sensations, emotions, and thoughts as they get pulled into the drama of the story. It can also be noted at this time that becoming better skilled at discerning sensations, emotions, and thoughts in the moment is one of the objectives of formal awareness exercises.

We then ask the large group to first share their physical sensations, then what emotions they experienced, and finally what thoughts they had. When asked to describe sensations, it is common for students to respond instead with a thought (e.g., I was anxious) rather than with the sensation (e.g., I could feel my heart racing). When this confusion between a thought and a sensation occurs, the teacher may point out the difference between a thought and a sensation and then ask the same student, "What did you feel in your body?" Another common confusion is the distinction between an emotion and a thought. In response to the question, "What emotions were you aware of?", some students may answer with "I felt that the surgeon should have recognized sooner that a tracheostomy should have been done." The teacher may respond back with the reflection that such a statement is not describing an emotion, but rather is the description of another thought. The student could at that point be asked again, "What emotion were you feeling?" while the teacher then remains attentive to see if the student is able to articulate a felt emotion (e.g., happy, sad, angry) rather than answering with the description of yet another thought.

Students may then be asked, "Which Satir stances (i.e., blaming, placating, super-reasonable, distracted, and congruent) did you see played out in the video reenactment?" At this point it may be helpful for the teacher to draw the diagram for each stance onto the whiteboard as a visual reminder. Students will likely note the possibility of many or all of the stances in the different actors. It is important to have students keep in mind the danger of labelling the stances of others and to point out that only the persons themselves can ultimately be aware of the internal conditions that result in outward directed actions. For example, while students may feel that many nurses in the video were in a placating stance, it is also possible that while their actions may look placating, the nurses may have decided that to confront the surgeon in the moment was not going to be effective and from their point of view being congruent meant doing what they tried to do (e.g., calling for an ICU bed).

The teacher may at this point want to make explicit the connection between an awareness of internal bodily sensations that we are purposively cultivating in our in-class GAP and suggest the idea that awareness of internal sensations (interoception) can be a useful source of information in clinical settings. The question could be asked to the large group, "If we had measurements of the hand sweat response of the people in the video what do you think we might have seen? Is it possible that many of them were aware, some even consciously aware, of what was going wrong but were rationalizing and or suppressing their physical sensations and thoughts?"

The teacher may then offer students a personal example of how they themselves have purposively brought their attention to a physical sensation, in the moment, to better listen to others or to make a better decision. An example for the coauthor (SL) is when using the hand sanitizer just outside a patient's room before entering, he brings his attention to the sensation of the liquid on his hands. The pause that this movement of attention away from the usual stream of thoughts and onto the physical sensation of the gel on hands creates allows him to return to the larger intention to enter the room open to whatever may await, rather than to stay with the default mode that would have him carrying in unrelated thoughts and issues from whatever he was doing or thinking before pausing to redirect attention. The same purposive bringing of attention to physical sensation may be helpful when, during a meeting of colleagues discussing emotionally charged topics, it can be easy to get "lost" in thoughts and the desire to interrupt can emerge despite the initial intention to not interrupt others when they are speaking. Noticing, in that moment, being physically halfway off the chair, attention can be brought back to the sensation of both feet on the ground, and a conscious choice can be made to reposition the body back to being fully seated. When mindful of body sensations, emotions, and thoughts, the primary intention not to interrupt is easier to recall, as is waiting for the other person to finish talking before speaking. When the decision is then made to speak, it is invariably with more calmness and effectiveness than if it had been as an interruption.

The field of aviation has defined situational awareness as "the processes of attention, perception, and decision-making that together form a pilot's mental model of the current situation" [7]. A more complete mental model would include not only paying attention to what is being observed from the outside (e.g., the oxygen saturation monitor alarm ringing) but also attention to internal thoughts, sensations (e.g., palmar hand sweat, racing heart beat), and emotions. Situational awareness is incomplete without the capacity to include internal thoughts, sensations, and emotions as sources of information about the current situation. In order to meet the challenge of maintaining awareness in demanding, stressful, unstable situations, we practice under much less demanding conditions while sitting in formal meditation. When learning to swim, it is wise to begin in the calm water of a pool in order to build up the skill to be able to swim in the turbulent water of the open sea. In a similar way, the skill of paying attention to both internal and external stimuli is practiced in the "relatively calm waters" of formal meditation in order to build capacity to maintain awareness in more stressful situations.

6. Mindful Movement

Mindful movement is introduced as another way to practice bringing attention to physical sensations during a series of sequential physical movements that the teacher leads the class by doing the movements while narrating the body positions as they are being done. The teacher stands, and we invite students to also stand up and form rows facing us so that they can see as well as hear the instructions. It is helpful to have students leave as much space as they can around themselves to avoid bumping into each other as much as possible. It is important to note to the students (and to oneself, as teachers may not be fully comfortable leading a "yoga-like" exercise) that what we are about to do together is neither equivalent nor intended to be equivalent to the kinds of instruction found in a formal yoga class. Rather, this is an exercise in purposively bringing attention to the body while it is in motion, in the same way we practiced bringing attention to the body and breath while seated at the beginning of class. It may also be helpful to point out that many students in the class will have more experience and expertise in yoga/mindful movement than the teacher leading the exercise. The point in articulating this is to anticipate the thoughts that may arise in students, such as "this is not the correct way to do a shoulder roll." It can be helpful to remind students that the purpose of the exercise is to focus on the quality of attention, rather than on their preexisting idea of the "correctness" of the position of their body during the exercise.

Students may also be reminded here that a lack of awareness was the essential factor missing in the medical error video and that the practice of purposively bringing attention to body sensations may be helpful when interacting with patients. As the teacher leads the class through the series of mindful movements (Appendix A), the teacher may also ask for attention to be brought to the "feeling tone," either pleasant, unpleasant, or neutral that occurs from moment to moment. Once the feeling tone is identified during a movement as either pleasant ("I like this") or unpleasant ("I don't like this") or neutral ("neither like nor dislike"), the instruction is to simply notice the arising and passing of these feelings as they change from one to the other. Students may also note how the desire for more ("I want") or for less ("I don't want") is associated with each feeling tone. When such feeling tones and desires are noticed, the idea is to note them and keep awareness open to the changing nature of sensations, thoughts, and feeling rather than "getting stuck" with wanting more or less.

The class can be ended while all are still in a standing position during the last mountain pose, and students are wished a good week. Students and teacher often both leave the class in a positive and energized mood.

See Table 5.1, Teaching template for Class 3.

Table 5.1 Teaching template. Class 3: Awareness and Decision-Making

Core concepts Awareness and medical errors Role of interoception in decision-making	Materials Medical error video Paper, pens, markers	Time Minutes
1. Guided awareness practice (10 minute; optional, "counting breath" method) Debrief: "Why do we practice these formal GAP exercises each class?" Define formal versus informal meditation		15
2. Check in "Has anything come up in relation to class last week, or so far in the course, that you would like to ask or talk about?" Offer to meet with students at their request either after class or at another time (offer your email/contact)		5
3. Awareness and medical errors Moving from Class 1 awareness of outer environment to Class 2 awareness of inner environment to today's class: Decision-making and medical errors Ask: "How common are medical errors?" (top 3–5 causes of death in the USA) Describe Iowa Gambling Experiment (draw 4 decks of cards on whiteboard)		15
4. Narrative exercise "Think of a time when you made an assumption, or jumped to a conclusion, and then later found out it was a mistake. For example, you may have felt a need to apologize to someone; or perhaps you realized later that you should have said something or spoken up when you had chosen to be silent." Give 6 minutes for writing Dyad discussion: A-B then B-A (3 minute each) for structured sharing of narratives Large group debrief: "How do assumptions (e.g., jumping to conclusions, biases) relate to decision-making?"		20
5. Medical error video (https://www.youtube.com/watch?v=JzlvgtPIof4) "Just a Routine Operation" Pre-video: "Notice 3 components of your experience while you watch the video: (1) Physical sensations, (2) Emotions, (3) Thoughts."		15
Debrief – questions to ask sequentially: "Describe your physical sensations during the video." "What emotions did you notice?" "What were you thinking?" (e.g., lack assertiveness, decision-making, communication, awareness of time, seriousness of situation, hierarchy) "What stances did you possibly see and to whom did you attribute them?" (review Satir stances on whiteboard) "Could awareness of physical sensations (including interoception) be a source of information that was missing or not used by those in the video?"		20
6. Mindful movement Transition to movement exercise by linking to second mind experiment (e.g., palmar sweat) and the video (awareness of body sensations: intero- and exteroception) Bring attention to the three possible "feeling tones" as they arise and fade away (pleasant, unpleasant, neutral)		10

References

1. Institute of Medicine. To err is human: building a safer health system. Washington, DC: The National Academies Press; 2000. https://doi.org/10.17226/9728.
2. Damasio A. Descartes' error: emotion, reason, and the human brain. New York: Penguin Putman; 1994.
3. Dunn BD, Dalgleish T, Lawrence AD. The somatic marker hypothesis: a critical evaluation. Neurosci Biobehav Rev. 2006;30(2):239–71.
4. Fukushima H, Terasawa Y, Umeda S. Association between interoception and empathy: evidence from heartbeat-evoked brain potential. Int J Psychophysiol. 2011;79(2):259–65.
5. Singer T, Critchley HD, Preuschoff K. A common role of insula in feelings, empathy and uncertainty. Trends Cogn Sci. 2009;13(8):334–40.
6. Bromiley M. Just a routine operation. 2011. https://www.youtube.com/watch?v=JzlvgtPIof4. Accessed 21 Aug 2018.
7. Endsley MR. Toward a theory of situation awareness in dynamic systems. Hum Factors. 1995;37(1):32–64.

Chapter 6
Class 4: Clinical Congruence

Tom A. Hutchinson

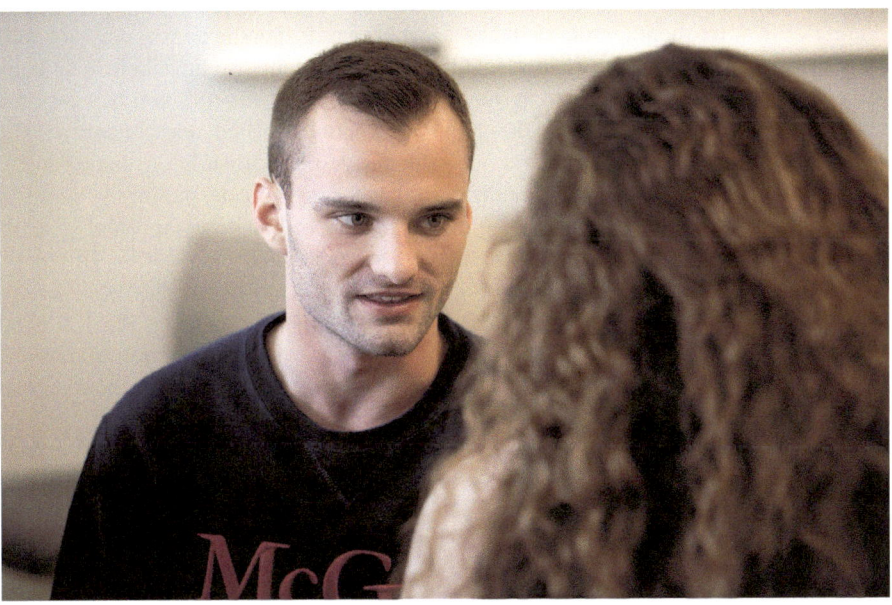

Fig. 6.1 Two students in a dyad

Overview

We wish to give students an experience and understanding of a key way of being that is central to effective clinical practice – clinical congruence when interacting with another person (Fig. 6.1). We begin by examining the particular characteristics of the clinical context, the stressors that are part of the clinical environment, and the

© Springer Nature Switzerland AG 2020   63
S. Liben, T. A. Hutchinson, *MD Aware*,
https://doi.org/10.1007/978-3-030-22430-1_6

unique job that physicians have to do in that context. We plan to give students an experience and understanding of how congruence can help them function effectively while caring for patients.

At this point in the course, we are beginning to know and have a sense of the different students in the class. Individual students begin to stand out and by this point we know all or most of their names. We have identified some students who appear very interested, some who appear to have an impressive level of insight, some easily distracted, and perhaps one or two students having a hard time or definitely resistant to what we are teaching. We believe this is an important time to employ our own mindfulness. Students who appear less interested are like distractions during meditation. They should not take too much of our attention and be blamed or pushed away; our job is to return our focus to what we are teaching.

It is also at this point in the course that we often begin to have a feel for this group of students as a whole and a sense of momentum in the group if things are going well. A frequent feeling in the first few classes is that the course may not work with these students. With any luck by Class 4, the students we have before us begin to displace the previous classes in our memories and our affections. It is a very real process of developing a new relationship that cannot be rushed, and our sense is that it is probably happening for us and our students at approximately the same time.

It is because of this phenomenon of a developing and deepening relationship over the seven classes of the course that we believe that it is important that one instructor or sometimes a pair of instructors teaches all of the classes. This is not always possible because of scheduling, and we do occasionally have one or two classes taught by another instructor. However, we do not believe it is ideal. It is not difficult for an instructor who sits in for only one class, but the overall relationship of the main instructor with the class can be affected in a way that robs the course of some of its depth for both the students and the instructor.

1. "Change Where You Sit in the Room"

We begin by asking students to change where they sit in the room. The purpose here is to change things in a way that may make some students uncomfortable but also more alert and aware. We may want to comment on the idea of "beginner's mind," which is a key ingredient of mindfulness. Changing position is a way of promoting this way of being.

2. Clinical Context

We begin by telling students we are going to look at what we learned in Class 2 (Chap. 4) on congruence and the communication stances in the context of caring for patients. We ask students to begin by individually writing down the characteristics of the clinical contexts they have experienced. These could be experiences they have had as students, or as patients, and can include contexts as diverse as ICU settings and outpatient clinics. Everything that they may have noticed – sights, sounds, smells, ambiance, and so on – is relevant. The aim is to put themselves back in that context in their imagination. We want that context to be present in their minds for later parts of the class.

We then transcribe, or have the students transcribe, some of the lists on the board. We may want to start with students who are relatively quiet, as a way of engaging them and ensuring they are heard. After the first list, we ask for additions from a second list and so on until we have a relatively complete picture, or the roughly 10 minutes for this part of the exercise is up. We may have some follow-up questions on particular items. For instance, if the students say the smell of the clinical environment, you may ask for more details, "What kind of smell or smells?" The purpose here is to get as full a picture as possible of what they have noticed. There will be commonalities in the lists of different students but also important differences that add to a more complete picture.

Once we have a list that is relatively complete, we begin to look at each of the descriptions and ask students which ones can induce stress. It turns out that most features of the clinical environment can cause stress. This may lead to a feeling of stress in the students, which is not a bad effect. It may make them more interested and open to hear about approaches that will allow them to function effectively in this stressful environment.

3. Bringing Together Satir Stances and Healing/Curing

We now turn the stress level up a notch by outlining the complicated job that physicians need to perform – curing and fixing the disease and facilitating healing in the patient. This conceptualization of medical care is something that we have already taught our students in first year. For those who are not familiar with this way of seeing medicine, we suggest that you read *Whole Person Care: Transforming Healthcare*, focusing on Chaps. 4 and 5 in that book [1].

We draw on the board the diagnostic process that separates the disease from the person and the resulting dual role of the physician to cure or fix the disease and to facilitate healing in his/her relationship to the patient as a person (Fig. 6.2). We then move towards a solution to the difficulties outlined by superimposing the congruence diagram on the physician, patient and disease diagram (Fig. 6.3) with the physician in the "self" segment, the patient in the "other" segment, and the disease in the "context" segment. We point out that clinical congruence is the overlap of congruence on the clinical context as shown in Fig. 6.3.

4. Review the Stances

We tell students that in this stressful environment, they are highly likely to unconsciously adopt one of the communication stances, which we ask the students to recall for us. It is important here to allow students to recall rather than simply

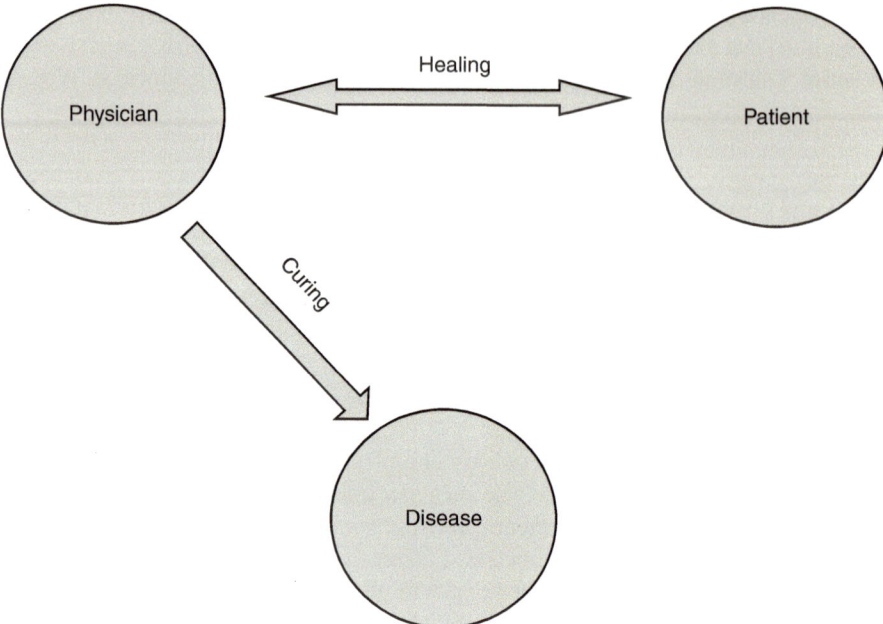

Fig. 6.2 Physician, patient, disease

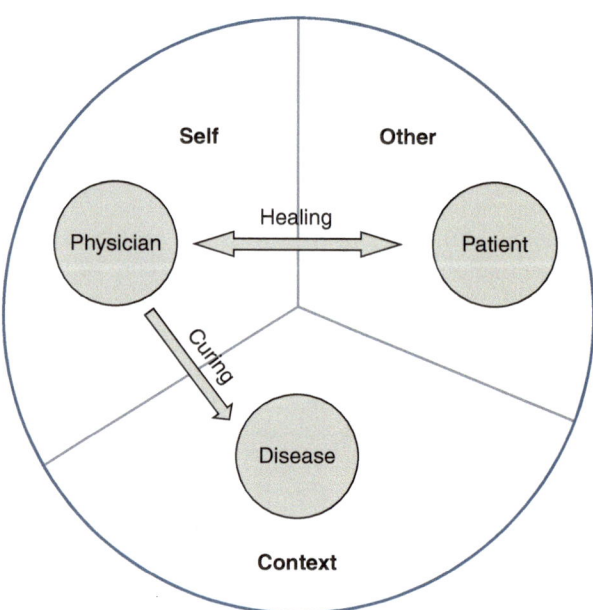

Fig. 6.3 Clinical congruence

supplying the information. We have sometimes found it helpful to ask specific students for a response to a particular question, such as, *"What is left out in the placating stance?"* This can help to include students who are not sufficiently engaged and tends to keep all of the students on their toes. We finish this section by pointing out that we will have a chance later in the class to see the stances acted out in a clinical situation to get a sense of how this works.

5. Awareness of "Soles of the Feet" Practice

But now we have a change of pace. There has been a lot of thinking and didactic teaching in this class so far. Now we want to give students an opportunity to move around and ground themselves in their bodies. The soles of the feet meditation has exactly that aim. Explain that we will be doing a meditation in which they will be standing with conscious awareness of their bodies and the sensations in their feet. This should not be done casually but with intention and attention to each moment as it unfolds.

Students are asked to stand up and notice the sensation in the soles of their feet as they sway slightly from side to side and forwards and backwards. We may then ask them to take a step forward with the right foot while leaving the left foot where it is in contact with the floor. They notice the changed sensations in the feet before returning the right foot to its original position. The same process is then carried out with the left foot. This should be a relatively short meditation with attention on the soles of the feet. We have found that this meditation can be easier than a conventional walking meditation because it takes less space in the room but, more importantly, because it tends to keep students more focused and aware. It avoids students walking relatively unconsciously and sometimes rapidly in a "business as usual," unmindful way.

This is a led meditation in which the teacher also does the meditation and issues simple instructions from time to time, such as "Notice your foot making contact with the floor" and "When you become distracted bring your attention back to your body and the soles of your feet." If you notice some students moving in a way that appears to you too quick or without attention, you may want to deliberately slow them down. At the end of the meditation, ask students to stop, pay attention to their body sensations, and then resume their seats.

We ask students what they have noticed. Some students may notice that this is easier for them than a focus on their breathing. We use this as an opportunity to point out that different approaches may work better for different people. They are free to experiment with what works best for them individually.

6. Embodying the Clinical Stances

This is the main focus of this class, and in many ways what has occurred earlier is simply preparation for this key part of the class. It is also an important part of the course in which we attempt to give students an experience of clinical congruence – the way of being that we hope they will bring to their clinical work.

You will need to have some familiarity and comfort with role plays to do an effective job of facilitating this part of the class. We do not believe that the expertise required can be obtained by reading or explanation. If this is not already part of your background, you will need some hands-on experience and probably some supervision. Since many medical schools now use role plays as part of their teaching, the required expertise may be available at your site. If not, you may want to consider enrolling in a program that provides such training.

We are not simply teaching a set of learnable steps or skills, although that is part of the process, but an understanding of ourselves and other people as positive and wonderful manifestations of what Virginia Satir would call "the life force." The underlying belief is that all of us, our students included, are good and looking for happiness and good experiences in life. This is more an act of faith than a provable fact, of course, but it makes a big difference in how we teach the course and particularly the part of Class 4 where we will do a role play using Satir's communication stances. This is not something that you tell students or discuss with the class but something that you need to remind yourself of as you get prepared for the role play. If this belief is difficult for you to completely take on, simply open yourself to this possibility for the duration of this class. The benefits to you and to the students will be significant.

Students will have a sense that this is a big moment and you should heighten the tension by explaining that the class will be acting out a clinical scenario and that you will be calling on individual students to play different roles. This is a time for the instructor to avoid casualness or laissez-faire and to bring the students' full attention and seriousness to the task at hand. Some students who get anxious or do not want to play a role may go to the bathroom at this point. This is not ideal, but there is not much that you can do but continue purposefully with the exercise. Do not call for a general bathroom break, as this will likely diffuse the energy of the group.

Now you proceed with picking the role players and conducting the role play. We will need six role players: one person to play the patient and five people to play five different physicians. We can ask for volunteers, which has the advantage that those playing the roles are keen to participate. Or we can pick role players arbitrarily, which allows us to include students who might not otherwise participate. At times we start with volunteers and then fill in the remainder with arbitrary choices. The two most important choices are the person who plays the patient and the person who plays the congruent physician, both of whom should be in your judgment students who will give the role their full effort and attention.

The specific clinical scenario that you use is a choice for you to make. We have found that it is important that the scenario discussed is serious and that the clinical approach to the problem is one that virtually all students would agree upon. One scenario that we have found works very well is that of a woman who has vascular complications of diabetes causing ischemia of her right leg. It has reached the point that her leg is unrecoverable and she needs an amputation to prevent the life-threatening complication of systemic sepsis. The interview that we play out focusses on the need for an amputation. The patient does not want the amputation and will do virtually anything to avoid losing her leg and suffering the resulting blow to her body image and self-esteem.

You are not simply watching but taking full control of what happens in the role play. Do not allow students who are observing the role play to make comments. There will be time for that later. Students may laugh at some of what happens, which is a normal way of relieving tension, but discourage an attitude of making fun of the whole thing. You will have to use your judgment in keeping the role play balanced and effective.

We begin the process by sitting the "patient" in a chair, giving her a card explaining her situation, and then giving any further information that she needs to play the role effectively. It is stressed that if something comes up about which she hasn't been instructed, she should simply make it up to the best of her ability. We then give a card to each of the role players playing a physician in one of the stances: placating, blaming, super-reasonable, distracting, or congruent. The front and back of each of the cards for the person playing the patient and for each of the physician role players are given in Appendix B. We ask the students to read the card but leave it on their seat when called on to play the role. We call on them in the order given above, giving each of them approximately 2 minutes to play the role. At the end of each role play, we ask the patient, "How did it go with this doctor?" If the final role play with the congruent student is going well, you may want to let that scenario go on a little longer. When all five roles have been played, you ask the audience to identify the stance of each of the physician actors. You then debrief each of the physician actors about their experience. You end with any final comments on his/her experience by the student playing the patient. You need to de-role all of the actors by asking them now to relinquish that role. They are free to retain whatever they have learned from the experience, but the role that they were asked to play was not them and does not say anything about them as persons or physicians. We end this part by giving the actors a round of applause.

As we do frequently throughout the course, we start the debrief of the role play by asking students in pairs to discuss with each other what they have noticed and what they have learned from the role play. In this dyad discussion, we do not pick an A and B and allow a free discussion for 5 minutes or so. We then debrief the role play with the full group. It is important here to focus on the insights that individual students have gained that may be relevant to their clinical practice. Comments on how good or bad the actors were or that they did not find it completely realistic should be listened to but followed by a question as to what they have learned. This can include the effectiveness of congruence but also comments such as that a particular stance may work very well. We agree with this and stress that it is not so much about avoiding stances but being aware when we are in a stance and making a conscious decision on how to proceed, which brings us to the last part of the class.

7. Introduce the Three A's: Awareness, Acceptance, and Action

We begin by asking students how they will avoid shutting down their awareness in their work. We use whatever comes up but stress that as human beings we have a tendency to move rapidly from awareness to action. For example, if I notice I am in a blaming stance and immediately take action to replace the missing part, the other person, in this case. We point out that there is another important step: to accept the situation and ourselves before we take action. This can seem counterintuitive and unhelpful, particularly if one is in a stance that is not ideal. There is fear that acceptance will make one less likely to change. We point out that the opposite is probably true, that real change is more likely to follow acceptance. Acceptance is not akin to resignation but a springboard for effective change.

This is an interesting discussion with students. Some students will embrace the value of acceptance before action; other students may feel that acceptance is giving in and will be very averse to acceptance. Your discussion of these ideas will also be affected by your own relationship to acceptance. For some instructors, and students, acceptance seems to go too far, and they are more comfortable with the word "allowing." You will likely not take students further than you or they are willing to go, which is fine. Whatever your point of view, the word "allowing" may be helpful for some students who have problems with "acceptance."

We follow this discussion by a short meditation in which students attempt to practice the three A's by focusing on their breathing. When they become distracted by thoughts or other sensations, they do not immediately rush back to focus on the breath but take a moment to accept their distraction before moving their attention back to breath. When the meditation is finished, you should dismiss the class without further questions or comments, which would simply take the edge off what has been learned.

See Table 6.1, Teaching template for Class 4.

Table 6.1 Teaching template. Class 4: Clinical Congruence

Core concepts Curing and healing in a clinical context Clinical congruence Awareness, acceptance, action	Materials Role play cards Paper, pens, markers	Time minutes
1. "Change Where You Sit in the Room" Students must also be next to new neighbors		5
2. Clinical Context "List what you have noticed in the clinical encounters you've had" Each student writes out a list Ask 2–3 relatively quiet students to write their own lists on the board		10
Have group participate together in deciding which words from the list are potentially stress-inducing, and then circle corresponding words from the lists written on the board		10
3. Bringing Together Satir Stances and Healing/Curing "In the clinical context physicians have challenging job, note many circled/stress words" Draw Fig. 6.2: "Need to attend to both diagnostic process and the separation of curing/fixing and healing at the same time" Draw Fig. 6.3: Clinical congruence – superimpose the self, other, context diagram		10
4. Review the Stances Draw out each stance Ask students to recall the four stances: "Which parts are left out in each stance?"		10
5. Awareness of "Soles of the Feet" Practice Much thinking thus far today; anchor attention to body sensation while standing		10
6. Embodying the Clinical Stances Set up scenario and pick students to play roles (patient "Karen" and five others) Give out role cards to players Seat "Karen" in a chair opposite the chair for the student playing the Satir stance For student playing "Karen," information on "who they now are" is on the card; tell students it is okay to make up additional information as needed For those playing physicians, each card has a diagram of the stance on one side and prompts on how to play that stance on the other side. "Read both sides of the card before going into role but put away your card during the role play." Run each role play interview for 2 minutes – follow each with a very short debrief of the patient Run the physician Satir stance role plays in order: 1. Placating 2. Blaming 3. Super-reasonable 4. Distracting 5. Congruent		30
General debrief of role play preceded by a dyad discussion		10
7. Introduce the Three A's: Awareness, Acceptance, and Action Ask: "How are you going to avoid shutting down part of your awareness in your work?" The reason to stress these three is that we frequently move too quickly from Awareness to Action without taking time to Accept (or Allow) what has happened		5
Practicing the three As: Sitting guided awareness		5

Reference

1. Hutchinson TA. Whole person care: transforming healthcare. Switzerland, Springer; 2017.

Chapter 7
Class 5: Building Resilience

Stephen Liben

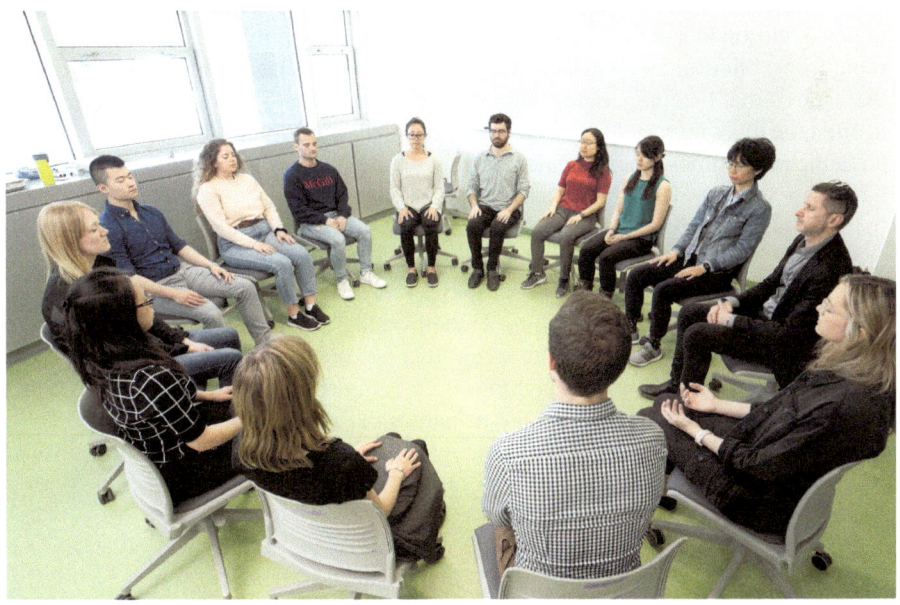

Fig. 7.1 Soundscape awareness exercise

Overview

Class 5, Building Resilience, is focused on awareness and deep engagement as sources of energy and inspiration that can be actively cultivated in the workplace as an antidote to the myth of "work-life balance" (Fig. 7.1). Rather than trying to balance what is called "work," with its implied negative, energy-draining connotations,

© Springer Nature Switzerland AG 2020   73
S. Liben, T. A. Hutchinson, *MD Aware*,
https://doi.org/10.1007/978-3-030-22430-1_7

with so-called life and its implied all-positive, uplifting energy, we acknowledge that much of our life is at work and that there is meaning and joy to be found within clinical practice work. The class also briefly explores the concept of burnout, and, while avoiding burnout is laudable, we feel it is important to emphasize that "not being burned-out" as a goal is aiming much too low. Rather than "trying to not be burned out," we aspire to clinical work that not only does not lead to burnout but even more so leads to being engaged in meaningful work where we find ourselves helping others while we grow into our own potential as more actualized human beings.

What we mean by "resilience" is not only the ability to rebound or recover after a disturbance but also the capacity to see each clinical encounter as a new opportunity to learn and to be helpful to the self and to others. The core experience of this class is the last one where dyads are set up for an exercise in deep listening. For this particular exercise, the ability of the teacher to be mindfully aware and to establish and maintain a slow measured pace is essential. The skill required to listen deeply is the same skill that is required in mediation awareness practice, that is, the ability to pay attention in a particular way. Deep listening is synonymous with, and inseparable from, mindful awareness. Once explicitly experienced students can know for themselves that listening, being fully present for another, is "doing something" and is often the most important, and the one thing, that is helpful for a patient, in particular at the many times where medicine cannot cure. In other words, after this class we hope that students will shift from seeing listening as "just" listening to regarding listening and being present as a crucial element in what they can offer their patients at any time and in all situations. Our hope is that students leave the exercise and this class with their own firsthand experiential knowledge of what it means to listen deeply and to be deeply listened to. Underpinning this is our own experience that within medicine doctors are more often than not poorly trained listeners, and that listening, which we see as synonymous with being fully present, is a skill that may be listed in the formal educational curriculum but is not necessarily valued within the informal and hidden curriculum.

1. Listening Meditation

The class begins with a 7-minute listening awareness exercise that focuses attention on the physical sensation of sounds (or on a selected piece of music) as they occur in the room. This "soundscape" is always available to awareness (we cannot close our ears in the same way we can close our eyes) and includes sounds that might be emanating from inside the body of the listener (e.g., the heartbeat) as well as those that appear from the outside. An alternative to bringing attention to the naturally occurring soundscape is to begin a breath awareness exercise as in previous classes and then begin to play a piece of music or a song. The onset of music would come as a surprise to the students who would have been expecting the same type of breath awareness exercise as in past classes. Whether the novelty of the unexpected music is beneficial to the awareness exercise or whether it inadvertently signals that novelty is desired when participating in awareness/mindful meditation is an open question that different teachers have different opinions on. Should a piece of music be played, it is important to emphasize in the debrief that liking or not liking the chosen piece of music is not the point. The learning point is rather to notice and be aware of preferences or aversions that may arise in response to the music. Some teachers may prefer not to introduce music with an element of surprise and instead inform students beforehand that a piece of music will be played and ask them to be aware of their "liking or not liking" or their being "neutral" to the music when it does appear. In the debrief, after a few students have commented on the "What did you notice?" prompt, it can be pointed out that mindful listening, reflected in student comments such as "I noticed that I liked/did not like/felt neutral about the music," means discerning how they feel rather than being judgmental about the content of the music/sounds.

How their experience during the soundscape exercise connects with clinical practice is the next question to raise with the large group. After students have initially responded, it can be pointed out that when patients tell the story of their illness experience (i.e., when a clinician is taking a medical history), each patient has their own type of illness narrative to convey [1], and some patient narratives are more "likable" and will resonate more with some clinicians than other types of narratives, in a similar way that some types of music are preferred over others. For example, there may be stories of illness that portray patients either as victims or as heroes. Clinicians may "like," "not like," or "feel neutral" about specific illness narratives (the hero narrative and war metaphors "battling against disease" are often the preferred narrative among physicians). The task is not for the clinician to deny to themselves their personal preferences/judgments but rather to be aware of spontaneously arising preferences for some types of narratives over others, as was practiced in the soundscape/music exercise. Bringing preferences/judgments to the clinician's conscious awareness, as in the internalized thought, "Now I am judging my patient's story," is reflection in action and increases the capacity to listen deeply even as likes and dislikes to what is being said arise. Without such a willful conscious awareness of likes and dislikes related to patient narratives, the danger is that clinicians will be less sensitive to, dismissive of, or not really hear less preferred or less likable patient stories.

2. Triangle of Attention

The teacher draws the Triangle of Attention onto the whiteboard (Fig. 7.2). The triangle describes how attention can be brought to thoughts, physical sensations, and emotions, the three aspects of subjective experience. While there is no agreed-upon answer to the question of the exact distinction between attention and awareness, for the purpose of this course, we define attention as the ability of the mind that can be willfully brought to bear on a subject or object that is present in consciousness. For example, if you are asked to bring your attention to the sensation of the palm of your right hand as you are reading this sentence in this moment, you

Fig. 7.2 The triangle of attention

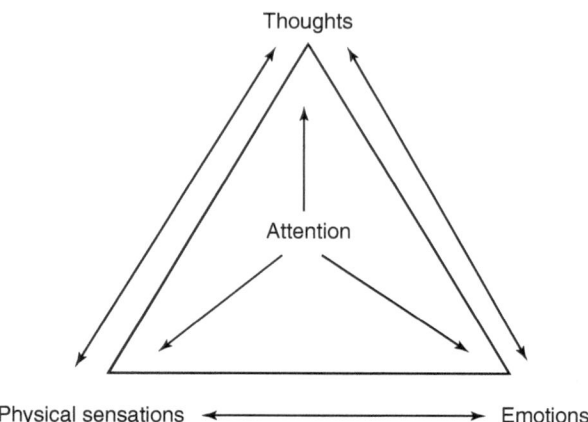

could then, if asked, articulate descriptions of these sensations as pressure, coolness, softness, hardness, etc. In that moment, the subject that you identify as "I" or "me" willfully focused attention on the sensations in your right hand in an analogous way that you could willfully point a flashlight in a dark theater towards a sound on a stage that you might imagine is in front of you. A flashlight being pointed in a dark theater towards the stage will illuminate only that which the circular point of light falls upon and little else. If one imagines a flashlight with an adjustable light beam that allows for a more narrow focused small pinpoint of light or a broadened wide diffuse spot of light, then in a similar way, attention can be narrowly focused as is experienced during deep concentration focused on one mental object, or as a wider focus of attention in what is often called "open awareness." Attention that is less focused and less intense would be a purposeful placement of attention that is still deliberate but not with the same intensity as during deep concentration. This type of non-concentrated, wider beam of attention is the type of willful attention that is being practiced in mindfulness exercises. It should be noted that other more concentrated types of awareness meditation practices exist in contemplative traditions, such as those that are intended to result in specific mental states that are not the subject of this course (e.g., the Jhana states in Buddhism).

If attention is akin to pointing a beam of light in a darkened theater, the emergence of awareness during meditation would be like a gradual increase in the overall illumination of the theater so that objects on and even off the stage that were previously in the dark would slowly have their outlines revealed until they became increasingly visible. In the dark theater, the flashlight could be pointed willfully to different areas of the stage in a similar way that *attention* can be instructed to be brought to bear on, for example, the sensation of the breath as air moves past the nostrils. This is opposed to *awareness* that is experienced in the dark theater as a gradual increase in the overall illumination that is not under conscious control, whereas where the flashlight points (*attention*) is under willful control. The gradual illumination of the dark theater would emerge as a result of pointing the flashlight in a specific way to specific objects on the stage. The increased visibility and discernment of different objects and activities on the stage is akin to the emergence of increased awareness as a result of focused attention awareness practice. The exact mechanism of how pointing attention in specific ways, as practiced in meditation, results in the emergence of a specific type of awareness (i.e., mindful awareness) remains unknown and is an active question in the neurosciences [2].

3. Define Mindfulness

Mindfulness can be defined in a variety of ways, but for the purposes of this course, the operational definition (a version of which was proposed by Jon Kabat-Zinn [3]) is offered to the students: "The awareness that emerges by paying attention in a particular way, that is non-judgmentally and with curiosity, moment to moment." The "particular way" that attention is focused also includes other attributes not listed in the formal definition of mindfulness like gentleness, trusting, patience, and non-striving.

The definition of mindfulness includes the words "in a particular way," which points to the *quality* of attention paid to specific objects like the breath or other bodily sensations. While it is important for the teachers themselves to know these qualities, how and when some of them are discussed in class will depend on what questions students are asking as the course evolves. The following qualities of mindful attention should not be lectured to the students, but rather the teacher may keep these qualities in mind to bring up in response to questions students may ask. Another way to teach the attentional qualities of being *nonjudgmental, gentle, curious, trusting, patient*, and *non-striving* is to ask students what they think is meant by each of these qualities.

Attention that is *nonjudgmental* neither suppresses nor denies any thoughts, emotions, or physical sensations that emerge in awareness. Should attention on the content of thoughts reveal a thought to be, for example, "I hate it when patients whine about their chronic pain," then being nonjudgmental would bring mindful awareness to then appreciate that thought is "just a thought" and is not necessarily true or helpful. The thought would be observed as it is but would not necessarily be believed as being true. Mindful awareness would see that the thought may or may not necessarily be true, and further evaluation might reveal the judgment implied in the word "whine" to be highly subjective, and it may say more about the limited capacity and prejudices of the listener rather than of the patient. Being nonjudgmental is not the same as not being able to make judgments or discernments. The brain will generate thoughts, such as "This is good, I like this" and "This is bad, I don't like this," in much the same way that the body produces heat and sweat during exercise. Being nonjudgmental means bringing awareness to these judgments as they occur in the moment and not necessarily believing them but rather holding them up for examination as in, "Is this really true or is this just my first, and not necessarily trustworthy, initial reaction?" Judgments will arise of their own accord in the same way that thoughts and emotions arise unbidden. However, once a judgment is noticed, once it is seen in awareness, the mindful attitude is neither to believe nor disbelieve the judgment but to hold the thought in awareness and keep it open to question.

Curiosity is the quality of mind that is interested in what is being sensed in awareness in the moment and welcomes what comes up in experience with an open gently inquiring attitude of "What is this?" Being curious goes with the attitude of "beginner's mind" – seeing things as if for the first time, without preconceived ideas. One way to introduce and practice the quality of curiosity in attention is to offer students the following instruction at the start of the first listening meditation of this class: "See if you can be curious about what you think, feel, and sense."

When, during a breath meditation, the awareness emerges that one is lost in thought rather than focussing on the breath, the *way* attention is brought back to the breath is with an attitude of gentleness. A useful metaphor is to think of bringing attention back to the breath in the same way you would carry a small bird back to their nest, gently but firmly, with *gentleness*, kindness, and compassion.

While attention can be willfully focused, like the beam of a flashlight, on thoughts, emotions, and physical sensations, the emergence of mindful awareness is dependent on conditions outside of direct control. It is no more possible to "make" oneself be mindful than it is possible to grow a tree from a seed by force. In the same way that growing a tree requires creating the necessary conditions, like preparing the soil, providing sunlight and water, and removing weeds, the emergence of mindful awareness is dependent on creating favorable conditions as practiced in meditation. The attitude of *trust* means trusting that mindfulness is an inherent quality that will emerge if the right conditions are created. An attitude of trust also means that while others can show you the steps to take, only you yourself can both do what is required and experience what there is to be experienced. Trust is needed for teachers pointing the way, and students must have trust in themselves to learn and grow. Trust is not so much the idea that "everything will work out" but rather that "I can learn from whatever comes up in experience."

While attention practices increase the possibility that mindful awareness will emerge, they do not guarantee its presence in any particular moment, and cultivating an attitude of *patience* is helpful. The feeling of impatience, of wanting to "see results" now, is itself something to be used in practice, to be held in awareness. Examining impatience with curiosity, with a gentle "what is this?" attitude, may reveal aspects of nonacceptance, of pushing away, or of an aversion to what is being experienced. Once recognized, there is the opportunity to consciously allow the feeling, the impatience, to be as it is and to follow with curiosity what happens next.

Non-striving means not trying to change whatever is already present, be it "wanted" or "unwanted" when it first appears in awareness. For example, the first reaction to being aware of being sad or angry might be to reject the emotion and immediately look for ways to feel "better." A mindful attitude or quality of non-striving would be to recognize the unwanted nature of the emotion and allow it to be as it is, to feel it as it is, before then choosing if, when, and how to respond in ways that might be truly helpful and not just mask or inadvertently replace the unwanted experience.

4. Burnout

Burnout as a concept is frequently referred to within the medical culture and is highly prevalent among healthcare workers [4]. The definition of burnout can be written onto the whiteboard and described as consisting of three components: (1) a felt sense of *emotional exhaustion* (e.g., "I just can't engage with other people's problems anymore"); (2) *depersonalization* manifested as treating people as objects and as "problems to be solved" rather than as whole human beings (e.g., the language that describes patients needing admission to a hospital as "hits" equivalent to bombs landing on a beach during war); and (3) a *lack of a sense of personal accomplishment*, feelings of incompetence, inefficiency, and inadequacy (e.g., "I feel useless, it all feels useless"). An additional aspect of burnout that helps distinguish it from the diagnosis of depression, with which it is related, is that unlike depression burnout occurs mostly at work and less at home. The large group is then asked to offer what they think the causes of physician burnout might be, and then either the teacher or one of the students scribes the responses on the whiteboard until there are about 10–20 possible causes listed. Once the list is complete, the large group is asked to identify which of the causes might be under the individual's personal locus of control, and each of these items is circled. Items that the group cannot agree on, causes that some think are under personal control and others think are outside of our control, can be circled with a dashed line.

The goal of bringing up the high frequency of burnout in medical professionals is not to scare students into thinking that "this will also happen to you," nor is it to normalize burnout as an expected outcome. The point is rather to have students see for themselves that while there is much in the external medical environment that could and should be changed (e.g., excessive paperwork and bureaucracy; the unacceptable intrusion of needing to enter data into a computer during the doctor-patient interaction in some healthcare settings; inequalities in access to care related to the way healthcare is funded), they do have choices in the way they respond to these challenges. Secondly, when students explore the factors that can lead to burnout and then identify the many that are invariably found to have an internal locus of control, they see that there is much they can do for themselves in the moment on the job to adapt to potentially burnout-causing stressors. In this way the teacher avoids "data dumping" the known high rate of burnout onto students with the resulting risk of activating feelings of helplessness (unhelpfully implying that burnout is an expected outcome of being a doctor). Instead, students see for themselves that they hold the power (agency) to modify many of the potential causes of burnout that are within their locus of control.

We propose that it is the way we respond that determines whether an experience is draining and depressing versus rewarding and energizing. Students are guided to appreciate this for themselves in the interactive exercise that demonstrates that the very same positive personality characteristics that are rewarded in medicine and in many other life domains, such as thoroughness, commitment, altruism, and being open to self-critique, when taken to extremes or in isolation, may instead function negatively and can lead to burnout and other undesirable outcomes. So-called good or positive personality characteristics are thus not seen as fixed entities, as being simply either or good or bad, but rather as existing along a spectrum from helpful to unhelpful that vary over time both within and between individuals. The teacher writes on the whiteboard a vertical list of eight "positive" personality traits consisting of thoroughness, commitment, perfectionism, questioning, altruism, caring, being rational, and being self-critical. The teacher then asks the large group, "What are possible negative, unhelpful, flip sides of these eight 'good' characteristics that can result from each of them being taken to extremes?" Each negative personality trait is then written on the whiteboard to the right-hand side of its corresponding positive trait. Groups typically find these types of pairings of good/bad traits:

- Thoroughness → Being over-compulsive
- Commitment → Boundary issues
- Perfectionism → Decision paralysis
- Questioning → Need for certainty
- Altruism → Neglecting personal needs
- Caring → Compassion fatigue
- Rational → Aloofness
- Open to self-critique → Overly self-judgmental

The group discussion on positive-negative traits is meant to evoke the understanding that resilience and avoiding burnout are related to a learnable capacity to be aware of our own unique personality traits rather than to the unhelpful idea that traits are fixed, that you either "have it or you don't." Personality traits are not seen as inherently positive or negative but may be helpful or unhelpful depending on whether they are balanced and used in appropriate circumstances. For example, the trait of being thorough is helpful when reviewing the medical chart of a complex patient but would be harmful if applied to analyzing the full differential diagnosis of a patient who becomes apneic where the immediate action of assisting ventilation is required. The trait of being rational is helpful in many circumstances related to the physician-disease (curing) relationship but may not be as helpful in the physician-patient (healing) interaction (see Chap. 6, Class 4: Clinical Congruence).

5. Define Resilience

Students in the large group are then asked, "What is your definition of resilience?". The definition we use is a person's capacity to functionally cope with and adapt to stress and adversity. Our concept of how to build resilience into medical practice is based on the following understandings:

- The skills needed to care for others, being patient, curious, and nonjudgmental, are the same needed to care for ourselves. In distinction to the concepts of altruism and self-sacrifice with their implicit zero-sum of having a cost to the caregiver for "giving care" to another, we see mindful resilience as helping both self and the other.

- Resilience as we define it has both fixed aspects specific to each individual, as well as learnable aspects that can be developed and improved with specific attentional practices. Fixed aspects are those character traits (e.g., those listed in Sect. 4. Burnout) that we may find especially true for ourselves that may not be true for everyone. For example, as a result of both genetic and environmental factors, an individual may find that questioning is a strong and often felt trait. Such a strong tendency to question, if unbalanced, may lead to a need for certainty that is unhelpful and impossible in most clinical situations where it is not possible to be certain of outcomes. While the trait of questioning might be considered "fixed" for that individual, the capacity to be aware of when it becomes unhelpful can be developed and strengthened.
- Being resilient is not the absence or elimination of negative thoughts and emotions. It is cultivating the capacity to *hold* unwanted thoughts, physical sensations, and emotions. What we mean by "holding" might also be described as developing capacities to *allow* what is unwanted without either denying or psychologically pushing away. We can allow what is unwanted to be as it is, as we know that with time feelings, thoughts, and sensations will inevitably change by processes not under conscious control. We also make a distinction between "allowing" and "accepting." Allowing is acknowledging the presence of mental states without the psychological action of attempting to alter or change the experience. Accepting, on the other hand, is the end result of a process whereby our relationship to what is initially seen as negative or unwanted, and has been allowed to be present just as it is, transforms from being negative to being neutral or even positive. The process of transforming the unwanted to a neutral or positive experience is not something that can be forced or proscribed – you cannot make yourself like or enjoy what was first experienced as undesired. However, what is under conscious control is the capacity to hold or allow what is unwanted or negative and observe as it evolves over time. When the evolution of the unwanted over time becomes seen or experienced as neutral or positive, it can be said to have been "accepted." Allowing is thus understood to be an actionable skill that can be practiced, while accepting is the end result of allowing and emerges of its own accord and in its own time.

The Resilient Zone Model (Fig. 7.3) uses the balance between the sympathetic and parasympathetic nervous systems to illustrate the resilient zone within which an individual has a healthy functional response to stress [5]. The two straight horizontal lines serve as the upper and lower limits within which lies the resilient zone. The resilient zone is where the autonomic nervous systems is well balanced and oscillates between relaxation and alertness. When the individual is activated by stress beyond their sympathetic nervous system's capacity to remain within the upper limit of their zone, they experience anxiety that may lead to panic or mania. The lower limit is defined by hypo-arousal, lack of energy, overwhelming fatigue, and an inability to act. The lower limit shares many of the attributes experienced in clinical burnout and depression.

Between the upper and lower limits lies the range of functionality within which a healthy individual may cycle up and down but always staying within the upper and

The Resilient Zone

In the "Resilient Zone" individuals have the best capacity for:
Flexibility and adaptability
Pro-social behavior
Executive functioning
Being responsive rather than reactive

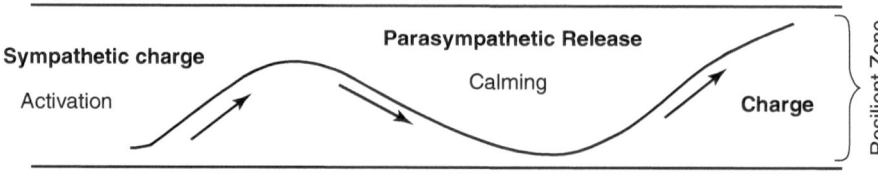

Individuals can learn to remain in and return to the Resilient Zone

Fig. 7.3 The Resilient Zone Model

lower limits. The frequency of oscillation of cycles may vary from minutes to hours to days to months. For many there are natural predictable changes in the flow of energy within a day and also within a week, month, or season. This may result in oscillations of energy that flow in shorter cycles of time (e.g., hours) that are embedded in longer cycles of time (e.g., within seasons or months), as cycles within cycles. For example, there may be times in the day when an individual feels more energized and able to perform creative or challenging work, and these periods of time may be embedded within longer oscillations that occur over months (e.g., seasonal changes).

The upper and lower limits that define the resilient zone have both movable and fixed aspects. The fixed aspects are resilient zone limits that are present at any one time, which are the sum total of genetic limits added to cultural/upbringing limits (nature and nurture). For example, individuals may have different hereditary thresholds before they feel anger in response to a stimulus. The "set point" for feelings of anger to emerge in response to a stimulus will not be identical between different people. There are also cultural and learned aspects to the upper and lower limits and in some cultures (and within some families) – behaviors are implicitly and/or explicitly encouraged as coping mechanisms when limits of resilience are reached. For example, there may be learned differences in the way an individual learns to cope with feelings of anger or panic. In some cultures, and in some families, when feelings of anxiety exceed the upper limit of the resilient zone, individuals may have learned to reach for alcohol, while in other families and cultures, the same stimulus (anxiety) may result in going to the gym to exercise.

The movable aspects of the resilient zone are those aspects that are amenable to change. For example, when working in a busy and stimulating medical environment, there may be a lack of awareness of such basic human needs as hunger (e.g., "Is it 2 o'clock already? I had no idea and I never ate lunch."). In this example, the upper limit of the resilient zone has been reached, but if there is a simultaneous capacity to bring awareness to the associated body sensations (e.g., tachycardia and abdominal sensations of hunger), behaviors can be enacted, like pausing to eat, to bring the person back into their resilient zone before they find themselves acting out undesirably and unhelpfully.

The key point of this model is to understand that we have control over our upper and lower resilient zone limits only if we develop our capacity to be aware of our thoughts, feelings, and physical sensations from moment to moment. This type of nonjudgmental moment-to-moment awareness (i.e., mindfulness) is itself a learnable skill that is cultivated with regular practice.

6. S.T.O.P. Exercise

S.T.O.P. (**S**top, **T**ake a breath, **O**bserve, **P**roceed) is a mnemonic for a specific type of informal awareness practice (definitions of formal versus informal awareness practices are given in Chap. 5, Class 3). We describe this informal practice as a "stealth" type of practice in that when S.T.O.P. is being done, no one other than the person themselves would be able to tell that anything was happening. The "S" in S.T.O.P. is the first letter in the acronym that also stands for the word stop itself. To stop means to intentionally create a break, a stop in the flow of automatic mindless thoughts and actions in clinical environments. Stopping can be so subtle an action that an outsider would not particularly notice anything, and the "stop" is behaviorally more of an internal psychological "stop" rather than an externally visible change in speed of movement. The "T" is for "Take a breath" and can mean to consciously take a breath, but it can also mean bringing attention to the breath you are already taking. We suspect that the reason why this popular mnemonic has "T" for "Take" rather than "A" for "Attend to the breath" is that S.T.O.P. is a better recalled mnemonic than S.A.O.P. The "O" is for "Observe" and means to bring attention, nonjudgmentally, to the felt sensations and then to thoughts and emotions that are present in the mind in the moment. The "O" provides the insight and discernment that is essential, for example, in the capacity to respond rather than react (as described in Chap. 4, Class 2). The "P" is for "Proceed" and is the ability to subsequently act from a new set point of mindful awareness rather than from the preexisting mind state of partial awareness or mindlessness. At the conclusion of S.T.O.P., actions taken are then based on mindful awareness, on responding, rather than on unconscious reacting.

Examples of S.T.O.P. in clinical medicine may include frequently experienced transition points, for example:

- Bringing attention to the sensation of water and soap while washing your hands before and after a clinical encounter
- Purposively focusing attention on the physical sensation of the doorknob (e.g., coolness, pressure, smoothness) when opening the door to a new patient encounter
- Paying particular attention to posture (becoming fully seated on the chair rather than sitting on only a portion of it as I just did myself while typing this sentence) and proper placement of the wrists and hands on the keyboard when typing on a computer
- Bringing attention to the sensation of the keys in your hand as you reenter your home at the end of the day. Allowing whatever thoughts are present to be known as they are

In order to show students what S.T.O.P. might look like in everyday practice and to help dispel the myth that S.T.O.P. might look strange in practice, the teacher can demonstrate entering a patient's room both with and without a mindful S.T.O.P., to have students see for themselves how S.T.O.P. can change the quality, tone, and rate of speech without changing the content of the first words spoken when greeting a patient. A student can be asked to play the role of a patient waiting to see the doctor. The teacher can first demonstrate a somewhat hurried and anxious physician entering a patient's room rapidly and saying, "Hello, my name is Doctor S," without making eye contact. The scenario is then repeated after a S.T.O.P., using the same words of introduction, "Hello, my name is Doctor S," but this time with a mindful pace that includes eye contact and nonverbal behaviors that embody presence.

At the close of this activity, students can be reminded that there are a host of different online applications that can serve as helpful reminders to use S.T.O.P. at either random or pre-planned times of the day.

7. Deep Listening Dyad Exercise

Students are now guided in a deep listening exercise that focuses attention on the story being told by one speaker to one listener within a dyad. In this exercise in paying attention, the primary task of the teacher is to set up the necessary conditions for students to be attentive and mindful as they listen deeply to one another. What we mean by listening deeply is the capacity of the mind to hear another person with mindful awareness (i.e., nonjudgmental, curious, gentle, patient, non-striving) of the words they use and do not use, the timbre of voice, pauses between words and sentences, and the nonverbal cues they embody but are not necessarily consciously aware of. Listening with mindful awareness also means being aware of our own internal thoughts, emotions, and physical sensations (the Triangle of Attention) from moment to moment and then using the skill of returning attention back to listening when thoughts have strayed from the speaker, in the same way that attention is brought back to the breath over and over again during formal meditation practice. The exercise of deep listening adapts the steps of pause, relax, open, trust emergence, listen deeply, and speak truth from Kramer's insight dialogue [6].

An essential component of this exercise is the energy level in the room before and during the exercise. Making a transition to this exercise from the S.T.O.P. exercise and demonstration that precedes it can be facilitated by a brief guided awareness exercise tailored to both the teacher's particular skill set as well as the felt energy level in the room at the time. For example, if the students are talkative and high energy, having them stand up and move through a brief set of guided movements, such as 2–3 standing mindful moving awareness exercises, may help to bring the energy level back down. Another option at the start of the listening exercise is to have students remain seated and have them focus their attention either on their breath or on the sensation of their feet on the ground. While the choice of which specific "attentioning" exercise is chosen is less important, what is essential is that the students begin the exercise at the optimal energy level – alert and awake but also relaxed and open, neither drowsy and inattentive, nor too anxious or excited.

Once achieved, the energy level of the students may need to be recalibrated during the exercise at key times, such as when switching roles between speaker and listener. What follows is one way to set up and guide the deep listening dyad exercise:

(a) Choose students to go into dyads so that they are paired up with the person sitting one space away (so that they are not paired up with the person next to them who they may have entered the class with and may have sat next to on purpose). Then, after reminding students to remain silent, have each dyad set themselves up facing each other.

(b) Check the energy level in the room, and engage in a large group sitting or standing awareness exercise as required to help them be alert and awake but also relaxed and open.

(c) Have students decide who will be A and B in the dyad.

(d) Give the instruction to A: "Think of a time when you experienced a difficult situation that challenged you (for example, a conflict between you and another person, a disappointment, a loss, a relationship betrayal) and that you found a way to cope with that was acceptable (more or less) for you. The episode may be a personal one or it may be in your role as a medical student. It may be ongoing and may not be fully resolved in your mind."

(e) Check in with students to be certain that all the A's have a story in mind by asking "Raise your hand if you have not yet been able to think of a story." If one or two students raise their hands (some students may have difficulty thinking of a past experience in the moment), the teacher can offer some additional tips to help, such as "Think of a time when you were last upset or unhappy with what you did or what someone else did, or perhaps did not do, that was disappointing to you." Encourage students to "Go with the first story that comes to mind. There is no need to avoid a story that you worry is not interesting enough."

(f) Offer guidance that when A is talking, B has a specific task as well. B is to listen, not to interrupt for any reason or ask any questions. If A runs out of things to say, then the dyad should remain in silence until the teacher signals that the exercise is complete. Remind them that A is to be doing all the talking and that B is to listen and not talk at all. Ask B to take particular note of the nonverbal body language of A as A tells their story.

(g) Have the group pause briefly again to bring their attention to their breath or to the sensation of their feet on the ground for about 30 seconds.

(h) Ask A to begin telling their story to B.

(i) After 5–7 minutes, most dyads will have stopped and will be in silence. Ask the remaining speakers to end their story, even if it is not complete, within the next 30 seconds.

(j) Guide the group in a brief awareness practice, such as feeling but not counting or assessing their radial pulse.

(k) Then ask B to tell back the story they just heard with as much fidelity to the words A used as is possible, such that B's first words might be something like, "I heard you say that ..." Only B should be talking at this time, and B should repeat what they heard back to A with as little interpretation as possible, avoiding phrases like, "I think you meant that ..." B should also include what they saw in terms of A's body language with phrases such as "When you started you had your hands folded, but when you talked about 'X' you had your hands open in front of you..." Allow 5 minutes for B to repeat back to A what they heard, including body language, as best they can.

(l) Before switching roles for B to become the story teller and A the listener, it may be helpful to have students stand up and silently change where they were sitting with their dyad partner, paying as close attention as they can to the sensations of their bodies as they move from one chair to the next (mindful movement) and very slowly and deliberately sit themselves back down into dyads.

(m) Repeat the steps above with the dyad instructions reversed so that A is now the listener and B is the storyteller.

In the large group, begin the debrief by asking, "What did you notice as the storyteller? Did it feel good, bad or neutral to tell your story?" Students often rate the experience as being positive or neutral. The next question to ask is, "What did you notice as a listener, was it pleasant, unpleasant or neutral, challenging, or easy?". The next question to explore then might be to ask how students felt when they had their story repeated back to them, whether they felt it was accurate and whether they were surprised by how well they were listened to. At this point, close to the end of this class, it may also be helpful for the teacher to point out what the students themselves may have already articulated in the large group debrief – that listening is active, it is doing something, it is not "nothing." You might ask students to think of who they would call if things in their life suddenly went very wrong. "Why would you want to call this particular person? Is it because they would have the answer to your problem, or is it because they would listen to you in way that would be helpful to you?" We underscore that the ability to listen is a skill that can be cultivated by mindful awareness. In the debrief, if students mention that it felt good to be listened to, the teacher can offer that speaking while being deeply listened to is energizing for both the listener and speaker, and therein lies the secret to resilience in clinical practice. Listening deeply to patients builds resilience and benefits both the patient and the physician. One antidote to burnout is deep engagement.

See Table 7.1, Teaching template for Class 5.

Table 7.1 Teaching template. Class 5: Building Resilience

Core concepts	Materials	Time,
Triangle of attention Resilience and burnout Deep listening	Music or song (optional) Markers	minutes
1. Listening Meditation "Soundscape" or piece of music Debrief – awareness of preferences (pleasant/unpleasant/neutral) and of sound as sound Ask: "How might this connect clinically?" "Patient stories as songs?"		10
2. Triangle of Attention Draw on whiteboard Flashlight onto thoughts, physical sensations, emotions Ask: "Why focus attention on body sensation/breath?" (sensations only felt now, less "sticky")		5
3. Define Mindfulness "The awareness that emerges by paying attention in a particular way, that is nonjudgmentally and with curiosity, moment to moment" (attention versus mindfulness)		5

4. **Burnout**
Definition on whiteboard: (1) emotional exhaustion, (2) depersonalization, (3) lack of sense of personal accomplishment (feeling incompetent, inefficient, and inadequate); occurs at work more than home
Student scribe; ask large group: "What are some causes of physician burnout?"
Circle causes we control; Ask: "Can we control lack self-awareness?"
Write eight "good" personality traits of medical students on whiteboard (left column); ask: "What are negative/unhelpful/flip-side of these characteristics?" (right column)
  1. Thoroughness ➔ Over-compulsive
  2. Commitment ➔ Boundary issues
  3. Perfectionism ➔ Decision paralysis
  4. Questioning ➔ Need for certainty
  5. Altruism/work ethic ➔ Neglect personal needs
  6. Caring ➔ Compassion fatigue (versus attachment to outcome)
  7. Rational ➔ Aloofness
  8. Open to self-critique ➔ Self-deprecation
		20

5. **Define Resilience** Individual's ability to properly adapt to stress and adversity. (1) Need to care for ourselves to effectively care for others, (2) can be developed, (3) capacity to allow space for all emotions and thoughts Resilient Zone Model: Draw Fig. 7.3 on whiteboard; "Zone borders are moveable" Ask: "What might affect the borders of the zone?" "What could you do to increase zone size?"		15
6. **S.T.O.P. Exercise** Demonstrate clinical example (e.g., pausing at door before entering room) Ask students to try using S.T.O.P. in coming week; mention mindfulness apps		10

(continued)

Table 7.1 (continued)

7. **Deep Listening Dyad Exercise**	45
"Think of a time when you experienced a difficult situation that challenged you (e.g., a conflict between you and another person, a disappointment, a loss, a relationship betrayal) and that you found a way to cope with that was more or less acceptable to you. Episode may be personal or in your role as medical student. Episode may be ongoing and not fully resolved."	

Engage dyads in slow process: pause, relax, open, trust emergence, listen deeply, speak truth

5–7 min.: instruct A to tell B their story (specify for listener B not to speak)

Use brief S.T.O.P. (e.g., "feel your pulse") between each activity

4 min. for the listener B to retell story to A and describe body language used

Repeat with B telling story to A and then A retelling story (or B–C if a triad)

Large group debrief: "What did you notice? First as 'listener,' then as 'storyteller'?"

Being listened to feels good (e.g., for a patient), is helpful, and is "doing something"

Being heard is, in and of itself, therapeutic and promotes healing

Deep listening is energizing and resilience building

One antidote to burnout is deep engagement

References

1. Kleinman A. The illness narratives: suffering, healing, and the human condition. New York: Basic Books; 1989.
2. Goleman D, Davidson RJ. Altered traits: science reveals how meditation changes your mind, brain, and body. New York: Avery; 2017.
3. Kabat-Zinn J. Wherever you go there you are: mindfulness meditation in everyday life. New York: Hyperion; 1994. p. 4.
4. Grunfeld E, Whelan TJ, Zitzelsberger L, Willan AR, Montesanto B, Evans WK. Cancer care workers in Ontario: prevalence of burnout, job stress and job satisfaction. Can Med Assoc J. 2000;163(2):166–9.
5. Leitch L. Action steps using ACEs and trauma-informed care: a resilience model. Health Justice. 2017; https://doi.org/10.1186/s40352-017-0050-5.
6. Kramer G. Insight dialogue: the interpersonal path to freedom. Boston: Shambala Publications, Inc; 2007.

Chapter 8
Class 6: Responding to Suffering

Stephen Liben

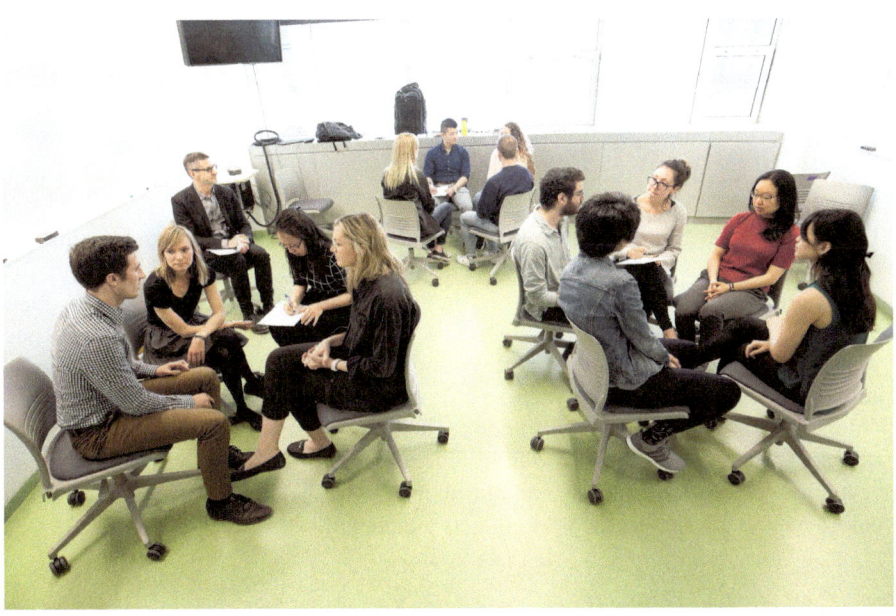

Fig. 8.1 Small groups creating list of helpful and unhelpful ways to respond to suffering

Overview

This sixth class has students explore different ways of responding to the universal experiences of pain and suffering that are either overtly or covertly embedded in patients' reasons for seeking medical care (Fig. 8.1). A subject that is rarely explored within the formal medical curriculum, how to respond helpfully to suffering, is an everyday challenge for clinicians. The etymology of the word "patient" comes from

© Springer Nature Switzerland AG 2020
S. Liben, T. A. Hutchinson, *MD Aware*,
https://doi.org/10.1007/978-3-030-22430-1_8

the Latin word for suffering. Patients, those who suffer, seek out medical care to help them feel better and eliminate, or at least reduce, their suffering. Experienced physicians know that the opportunity to easily and rapidly resolve the cause of a patient's suffering, that is to cure, is rare and that most of their work will instead be to seek out ways to help patients suffer less. For chronic illness where cure is neither possible nor expected, the goals of care shift to reducing pain and suffering as well as helping patients adapt to their "new normal." By this penultimate class of the course, building upon the 10 hours of small group work done over the past 5 weeks, enough of a trusting small group dynamic has been established to help students navigate the deep waters of responding to human pain and suffering. This class can have a strong emotional impact on students and in their course evaluations they frequently write that they found this class in particular to be both memorable and helpful. We have found that student learning and growth take place best when students are able to be challenged not only cognitively, but also emotionally, and by this class students are well prepared to reflect on emotionally challenging issues such as personal mortality.

1. Guided Awareness Practice

The class starts with a 10-minute guided awareness practice (GAP) that begins with either a breath awareness or a body scan and ends with attention focused on internal and external sounds, the "soundscape," in the last few minutes. While paying attention to the internal and external soundscape, students can be prompted to notice how sounds arise and pass away on their own and that once a sound fades away, it cannot be heard again. Attention may also be directed to asking if they are able to hear "sounds as simply sounds" and to notice the layers of meaning and judgments that so quickly get attached to any sound as in, "Oh, I like (or hate) that sound." It may be helpful to ask, "Can you hear sounds that arise on their own as the raw sensation, before meaning and liking/not liking gets attached?"

2. Pain and Suffering

The large group is asked to offer their understanding of the definition of pain and of suffering and how they differentiate between the two concepts. Students are then asked to think of examples when physical pain may not be associated with suffering. Students typically answer that the pain of child birth is an example of pain without suffering. Asking "What is suffering?" leads to a discussion of the distinction between what happens and the reaction to what happens in the chain of events that leads to experiencing suffering. A key concept is the understanding that while physical, emotional, psychological, and social pain are an inevitable part of the human experience, how we respond to what happens, as opposed to what happens per se, can make things better or worse and makes all the difference. Being human means to have a body that breaks down and feels aches and pains. While pain is inevitable in life, there are types of suffering that are optional. Almost 40 years ago, Eric Cassel wrote about the relationship between illness and suffering and made the important distinction that suffering occurs by persons, and not simply by bodies [1]. Cassel described suffering as an experience that results from any threat to the intactness of a person, and he helped define "persons" as complex social and psychological beings.

Pain is the initial reflexive unpleasant physical or emotional experience that occurs when we either get what we don't want (including physical pain and other symptoms) or don't get what we do want (including wanted states of mind such as feeling peaceful or calm). Suffering, on the other hand, is what we add to the pain that arises; suffering is how we relate to our pain. Suffering is the result of the story we tell ourselves when we are experiencing pain. It is this additional story that makes things worse for us that leads to suffering. For example, when a new physical sensation of pain is felt in your shoulder and you are an otherwise well 25-year-old woman who lifts weights at the gym three times per week, thoughts will arise, such as "I must have pulled a muscle in my last workout – I need to adjust my weight training next week." If, on the other hand, you are a 50-year-old woman who was treated for breast cancer 2 years ago and you get the identical sensory sensation in your shoulder, your thoughts might be, "Oh no, I hope this is not the cancer coming back…I don't think I can take another round of treatments again…I just can't go through cancer again!" The physical sensation felt in the shoulder as pain may be identical in the 25-year-old and 50-year-old and is an inevitable part of life. The story that is added on, the narrative created around the sensation of pain, is what leads to suffering. It is the narrative "add on" that is the extra unnecessary aspect that turns a physical sensation into suffering, and it is this narrative that is open to cognitive re-evaluation. When the storyline that is added to the painful sensation is seen for what it is, simply a narrative that is not necessarily reflective of reality and is not necessarily a true or helpful story being told by ourselves to ourselves, the possibility for reinterpretation of the story and lessening of suffering occurs [2–4]. The possibility of reducing suffering in reaction to physical pain is also possible for emotional pain. When a painful emotion is first experienced, such as grief after the death of a loved one, there inevitably arises a storyline, a series of thoughts, that is added on to the initial emotional pain. Thoughts about emotions, such as "I will never get over this painful feeling of grief and loss and I will always feel like this," are cognitive errors (we tend to overestimate how long we will feel negative emotions) that can prolong grief and complicate bereavement [5].

Another way of understanding suffering is that beyond the raw experience of pain, suffering results from the resistance to pain, in the form of the stories we tell ourselves about why we should not be feeling what is already happening. Suffering is the product of pain multiplied by the resistance to experiencing pain, analogous to the following formula:

$$\text{Suffering} = \text{Pain} \times \text{Resistance}$$

In this equation pain is not under conscious control, pain simply happens, but how pain is resisted is within some cognitive control. If resistance to pain is reduced, then while the sensation of pain remains, the experience of suffering is reduced. While acceptance may be the opposite of resistance, acceptance is the outcome of a process and cannot be willed. We cannot "decide" to stop thinking specific thoughts or feeling what we are feeling. What we can do, what is under cognitive control, is develop a capacity to allow unwanted thoughts and feelings to be, rather than to actively find reasons why they should not be present at all. To allow is to recognize the pain for what it is and allow its presence to be felt as it is. In other words, to be okay with not feeling okay, instead of the reflexive pushing away and resisting of the painful experience that is already there. It is the not allowing, the resisting, that itself is the fuel that feeds the fire of suffering. When unwanted thoughts and feelings are able to be held in consciousness, to be allowed, over time they may be accepted.

Once the concepts of pain and suffering have been discussed, students are guided to an exploration of suffering that extends to the broader domains of suffering beyond pain and the medical setting. Students can be asked, "Besides physical pain what are some other ways that suffering results from the stories we tell ourselves about who we are, what groups we belong to, and what matters in our lives?" The examples students offer can then be grouped into the different domains of suffering that include social (exclusion), economic (poverty), existential (loss of meaning), and religious (loss of faith).

3. Helpful Versus Unhelpful Responses to Suffering

The class is now divided into four smaller groups of 4–5 students each with one student per group assigned to be the scribe. Two of the small groups are asked to create a written list of "helpful ways to respond to suffering," while the other two small groups are asked to create a list of "unhelpful ways of responding to suffering." Prompt students by having them "think of a time when you were suffering in some way, when something in your life was not going well. Think of your interactions with other people at that time. These two groups make a list of what helped and the other two groups list what did not help."

After about 10 minutes, ask one person from each group to write their group's list on the whiteboard so that all the helpful ways to respond are on one side of the board and all the unhelpful ways are on the other side. As you review the lists with the large group, ask for clarifications when indicated (e.g., "Can you say more about what is meant by 'ruminating'?"). As always in this course, the teacher may choose to elaborate on points raised or not raised in the lists. For example, in one particular class, the unhelpful list included the term "giving up," while the helpful list had "surrendering." Asking students what they meant by these two terms led to a conversation of the difference between giving up and surrendering. Giving up was found to have elements of resignation and pushing away unwanted thoughts and emotions, while surrendering had qualities of allowing and accepting (without necessarily agreeing with or validating) what was already occurring in experience.

Students next can be asked, "What is the connection with these two types of lists and the Satir stances?" Typically, what is noticed is that unhelpful behaviors fit in well with non-congruent stances, while helpful actions often fit best with the congruent stance. Students can then be asked, "How could you yourself move to embodying more helpful ways of responding to suffering?" One way to move out of unhelpful non-congruent Satir stances (blaming; placating; super-reasonable; disorganized) to the more helpful congruent stance is to bring back to awareness what is missing. For example, when the awareness emerges that we are in a blaming stance, to become more helpful would be to include in awareness those parts of the other person's experience that were being left out.

4. Awareness of Time Exercise

While the individual steps needed to lead this exercise are quite simple, what is essential is for the teacher to be fully present themselves and to mindfully and deliberately set the tone and pace of this emotionally intense activity. The tone to aim for is one where students are settled in body and mind to deeply engage with the progressive imagining of less and less time left to live. Pacing and setting the tone are affected by inserting brief mindful awareness exercises as needed. It is not uncommon to see some students tearing up by the end of this exercise.

Each student is provided with a pen and paper and is asked to reflect on the following question by themselves and in silence: "Think of 4-5 important goals and/or dreams you are pursuing in your life and write them down in list form. You will not need to share this list with the large group, and when you are asked to share in a dyad, if there is something specific on your list you are embarrassed to share (such as your private dream to become a rock star!) then you will have the option to not bring it up." The example of dreaming of becoming being a rock star (or other fantastical dream) is deliberately mentioned as it implicitly gives permission for students to write on their list what they really are dreaming of, even if it may be unrealistic.

Once students have created their lists (after about 5 minutes), they are given a few minutes to share their lists in dyads. The next step is to have them move out of their dyads and sit by themselves again and if necessary to refocus their attention with a brief GAP (such as bringing their attention to their feet on the floor or to the sensation of their radial pulse). We then ask students to look at their lists but this time to imagine that they now only have 6 months left to live. "With only 6 months left to live, you know that you will not be alive in [insert name of seventh month].

What would change on your list? What would remain the same? Please add or delete what you need to make a list of dreams and goals if you had only 6 months left to live." After a few minutes, have them again share these modified lists in the same dyads. When the dyads are complete, have students, again on their own and after another GAP if required, look at their list again, but this time imagine that they have only 1 month, only 30 days, left to live. We then ask, "What do your lists look like now, and what do you need to modify add or subtract with only 30 days left to live?" We then again have students share this modified list in their dyad for a few minutes. Finally, in the last part of the exercise, we have students reconsider their list while imagining that they have only 1 day, only 24 hours, left to live. They again share this final list in dyads for a few minutes.

The teacher then reconvenes the large group to discuss, "How did your list change with less and less time left to live? What was on your list with only 1 day left to live?" Students most often say they had "being with family and friends" on their 1 day left to live list. When time left to live is very limited, what often emerges is that it is relationships and simply being with others (as opposed to doing or acquiring things) that we care most about. Students find an increased appreciation for the importance of relationships that they already have and have had all along. Another possibility is that they might express how easy it was to let go of many goals or how longer-term goals that previously might have seemed absolutely essential to their happiness were found to not be so important when their time was limited.

Students are then asked, "How might this exercise relate to patients you will be caring for?". What often emerges in group discussion is that some patients face the sudden reduction of life expectancy when given the diagnosis of a life-threatening illness. For these patients this exercise is not hypothetical but is a reality that they live out in real time. Students may also gain a deeper understanding that what they themselves found really mattered for them, such as the importance of close relationships, is also true for many patients facing the real situation. The discussion might also include the possibility that in their role as physicians, they themselves may become an important relationship to their patients with life-limiting illness. The lived experience of this exercise, coupled with the deep listening activity of the previous class, is intended to have students feel for themselves that there is always more that they can do for their patients, even those that have a fatal incurable illness, as long as they understand that *being with* their patients is not only "doing something" but is often the very thing that is most needed and helpful. We have found that to be with another person who is suffering and in pain is a learnable ability involving regulating one's own emotions and discomfort. Having the ability to practice mindful awareness in the presence of another's suffering allows for "staying with" and "allowing" the uncomfortable emotions that may be evoked and leads to desired helpful responses instead of unhelpful reactions. Physicians who can bring mindful awareness to being with the pain and suffering of their patients are not learning to just tolerate pain; they are creating the conditions for compassion to emerge in themselves [6]. Such mindful compassion is energizing, bringing agency and purpose to the physician who can see for themselves that their mindful presence is helping to reduce their patients' pain and suffering. This agency, this learned capacity to be with and reduce pain and suffering, brings meaning to clinical work and is an antidote to burnout.

5. Terror Management Theory and Mortality Salience

The awareness of time exercise just completed had students think concretely and explicitly about their own mortality. Such a raised conscious awareness of one's own mortality is termed "mortality salience" (MS) in terror management theory (TMT) [7]. The teacher then explains TMT and offers examples using some of the studies and explanations of TMT outlined below.

Mortality salience is increased by much subtler interventions than being asked to think about our own death (as was just done in the awareness of time exercise), such as being interviewed in front of a cemetery or funeral home or after subliminal exposure to the word "death." In these less obvious situations, people are not consciously aware that their MS has been raised, but nonetheless their actions and subsequent decisions are still affected. The teacher can offer an example of a study that had two groups of Christian American medical students read case histories and then rank the medical risk of patients with complaints of chest pain who presented to the emergency room [8]. The medical case histories were identical, with the same signs and symptoms, except for either a Christian-sounding name and identified religion or a Muslim-sounding name and religion. Before reading the case histories and then deciding on the extent of medical risk for each patient, one group of students had their MS raised by filling out a questionnaire, while the other control group filled out a non-MS raising questionnaire. Although the two groups of Muslim and Christian patients had identical symptoms and risk factors on presentation, students that had their MS raised assigned greater medical risk to the Christian patients when compared to the Muslim patients. The authors concluded that the medical students with raised MS unconsciously reduced their death anxiety by assigning patients who seemed more like them (Christian) to have a higher risk and therefore requiring more intensive investigation and treatment when compared to "others" (Muslims), who had identical medical presentations but were outside their own social group.

In TMT mortality salience is the cause of existential anxiety that is unconsciously reduced by the person attaching themselves more closely to their own cultural group identity and distancing themselves from others that are perceived to be outside their group. Such group identity includes religion, race, gender, and other socially constructed groups that individuals self-identify they belong to.

According to TMT, when MS is raised, a person becomes anxious and unconsciously decreases their anxiety by more strongly identifying with their own group
identity (e.g., race or religion), thus bolstering their worldview and self-esteem.
This unconscious psychological defense mechanism may partly explain how racist
behavior emerges, as more closely identifying with one's own culture means that
other cultures are seen as threatening. In medical settings, physicians' MS is raised
on a regular basis in their day-to-day interactions with ill patients who starkly manifest human vulnerability to illness and death. Physicians who identify with medicine as a group culture may unconsciously see ill patients as outside of their own
medical culture, as the "other."

One possible consequence of unconscious "othering" of patients was demonstrated in a study where terminally ill patients presenting with a critical illness who
had previously repeatedly articulated their desire for palliative care over life-
prolonging treatments were nonetheless encouraged by medical students (who had
their own MS raised) to accept aggressive treatments as a way to decrease medical
students' fears of their own mortality. That is, only the students who had their MS
raised (compared to a control group that did not have their MS raised) encouraged
patients to accept aggressive medical interventions. Most importantly, after working
in a palliative care clinical setting, students with increased MS no longer encouraged support for aggressive medical interventions in terminally ill patients with
preexisting expressed wishes against life-prolonging interventions [9]. In palliative
care, death and dying are seen as difficult but normal experiences, as opposed to the
idea embedded within much of non-palliative care medical culture, that to be ill and
die is to fail. Students who spent time working in palliative care had the opportunity
to openly discuss and resolve some of their anxieties concerning death and dying,
supporting the notion that the unconscious effects of raised MS on decision-making
may be decreased when brought to conscious awareness. When we are unaware that
our MS has been raised, we act out unconsciously to reduce our anxiety in ways that
elevate our own social group and lower others. However, when we become aware of
the anxiety that results from having our MS raised, we can consciously choose to act
in ways congruent with our values of inclusiveness and equality instead of out of our
unconscious fearful self-identity that vainly grasps for certainty in an uncertain
world.

Group discussion is then oriented to asking questions to elicit from students the
understanding that it is their capacity to be aware that is central to avoid being
caught in unconscious and unhelpful reactions. The group can be prompted to look
at the list of helpful and unhelpful ways to respond to suffering that was put onto
the whiteboard earlier and asked, "How might you shift from unconscious MS
based behaviors to greater awareness and more helpful conscious responses to suffering?" Students who respond to the question with the answer, "We need to be
more aware," can be asked, "How can you be more aware?". A discussion of how
to increase awareness, other than simply saying to oneself, "I need to be more
aware," can ensue and often leads to the conclusion that setting an intention to be

more aware is not sufficient to produce behavior change. Knowing how important it is to be more aware is not enough to make any of us more aware more often, in the same way that knowing the importance of being calm and not panicking in a medical emergency is not enough to ensure appropriate behavior when the emergency really occurs. What is done in practice to increase the chances of not panicking in medical emergencies is that courses are given (e.g., advanced life support courses in medical education) that simulate emergencies as a way to practice in a safe and controlled setting, over and over again, how to better respond when the actual emergency takes place. What students may find is that increasing their capacity to be aware when their MS is raised requires both the intention to increase their awareness coupled with a commitment to a regular awareness practice.

6. "Just Like Me" Guided Visualization Exercise

Adapted from the Buddhist practice of "metta loving kindness," this GAP uses the students' developing skill of stabilizing attention on the breath that has been built up with previous guided awareness exercises to help create the conditions that make prosocial attitudes, such as empathy and compassion, more likely to emerge [10]. While, on one hand, directives to "feel compassionate towards self and or others" are clearly ineffective (in the sense that emotional states can no more be willed into existence than commanding someone to "relax" would result in feeling relaxed), it is, on the other hand, possible to help create the internal mental conditions that promote an increased possibility for empathy and compassion to arise.

The guided awareness exercise begins by focusing attention on the sensation of the breath and then proceeds to ask students to visualize in their mind's eye a person or being (it could also be a pet or a person who is no longer alive) that they feel positively about, a person that has been supportive and helpful. When such a person has been visualized or imagined, the teacher states that phrases will be said aloud that are meant to be silently internally repeated and directed towards the helpful person that has been brought to mind. Mention might be made that there is no expectation that the words themselves need generate any specific thoughts or emotions and that whatever is being thought or felt at the time is simply acknowledged and held in awareness without judgment. The phrases are then verbalized aloud by the teacher:

- *This person has been sad, disappointed, angry, hurt, or confused, just like me.*
- *This person has experienced physical and emotional pain, just like me.*
- *This person wishes to be free from pain and suffering, just like me.*
- *This person wishes to be safe, healthy, and loved, just like me.*
- *This person wishes to be happy, just like me.*

After a minute or so, the teacher suggests that attention be redirected back towards the sensation of the breath. Students are then invited to bring to mind a neutral person, someone that they do not know well, who may be seen only from time to time and for whom there is no association with any especially positive or negative feelings. Such a person could be a bus driver or a person who works the counter at a store, for example. Once this person has been called to mind, the five phrases are repeated aloud and directed towards the neutral person with the same sequence of pauses and attentional instructions as in the first visualization. The process is then repeated for a person that is regarded negatively, someone who has done harm to us or has been a "problem" and whom we dislike and can easily state several reasons why.

After the three sets of visualizations of a positive neutral and negative person/being are completed, the large group is debriefed by asking, "What did you notice?". In the debrief, students may comment that they found it hard to "forgive" the person they felt negatively about in the last visualization. Students can be reminded that there is no need or intention to forgive but rather to simply acknowledge the common human desire to be safe, healthy, and happy. The fact that the way individuals act in the world to feel safe and healthy and happy can result in increased suffering for others is also true. The point is neither to forgive nor condone the harms that others have inflicted but is instead to bring to conscious awareness the commonality of goals we all share, in order see the "other" as human, as "just like us", albeit with different, and sometimes dysfunctional ways of reaching towards the same goals.

This exercise rests on several premises that remain to be further investigated and proven. The first premise is that we are more likely to feel and act positively towards someone who we perceive as being similar to us, who is "just like us." The opposite of feeling positively towards those we see as just like ourselves would be the dehumanization, the "just not like me" shift in judgmental attitude that occurs as an essential step in objectifying others. The second premise is that when specific thoughts, feelings, and emotions are present, feeling and acting with compassion are more likely to occur. In other words, when the thought "I am just like this other person" is coupled to the emotion "I am feeling open and secure," the likelihood that hate is also present at the same time is very low. The third premise is that cultivating specific aspects of mind, such as compassion, builds up an increased propensity and capacity to have that same mind state emerge more often. There is some evidence to suggest that mindfulness practices result in structural changes in the brain, while there is less evidence on its impact on successfully increasing prosocial behavior [11].

See Table 8.1, Teaching template for Class 6.

Table 8.1 Teaching template. Class 6: Responding to Suffering

Core concepts Pain versus suffering Being with and responding to suffering	Materials Paper, pens, markers	Time, minutes
1. **Guided Awareness Practice** 10 minutes, end with soundscape Debrief: "What did you notice?"		15
2. **Pain and Suffering** Ask: "What is pain? What is suffering? When is physical pain NOT suffering?" Offer: Suffering = Pain × Resistance Six domains of suffering: physical, emotional, social, economic, existential, religious		10
3. **Helpful Versus Unhelpful Responses to Suffering** Four small groups of 4–5 students each create written list – two groups create "helpful" list and two create "unhelpful" list "Think of a time when you were suffering. These 2 groups make a list of what helped and the other 2 groups list what did not help." One student in each group to whiteboard: two columns (helpful and unhelpful) Large group discussion: "How does this relate back to Satir stances?" (Hint: bring in missing part of non-congruent stance)		20
4. **Awareness of Time Exercise** "List (by yourself) 4–5 important goals/dreams you are pursuing." Then share list in dyad Reduce time left to live to 6 months, 1 month, 1 day, and have students revise list each time the duration of life left changes and briefly discuss again in dyads Debrief as large group: "What was on your 1-day-left list?" (outcome = mostly shared values of being with loved ones as time becomes shorter) Ask: "How does this relate to patients (sometimes it is their literal experience)?"		20

5. **Terror Management Theory and Mortality Salience**
Explain: Culture and self-esteem as defenses against unconscious death anxiety; MS is raised by asking people to think about their own death, fill out life insurance forms, or be interviewed in front of a cemetery
Ask: "What is link between awareness of time exercise and the clinical setting?"
    Christian medical students in cardiac risk ER study
    Students and palliative care rotation
Refer back to list on whiteboard of helpful/unhelpful responses to suffering.
    Unconscious MS shifts us towards unhelpful response to suffering, and conscious awareness shifts us towards helpful responses
    Ask: "How might it be possible to shift from biased unconscious MS based behavior to greater awareness and more helpful response to suffering…?"
Ask: "How can you increase your awareness in clinical practice?"
		15

6. **"Just Like Me" Guided Visualization Exercise** Progression from positive, to neutral, to negative person Debrief: "What did you notice?"		10

References

1. Cassel EJ. The nature of suffering and the goals of medicine. N Engl J Med. 1982;306(11):639–45.
2. McCracken LM, Gauntlett-Gilbert J, Vowles KE. The role of mindfulness in a contextual cognitive-behavioural analysis of chronic pain-related suffering and disability. Pain. 2007;151(1):63–9.
3. Veehof MM, Oskam MJ, Schreurs KMG, Bohlmeijer ET. Acceptance-based interventions for the treatment of chronic pain: a systematic review and meta-analysis. Pain. 2011;152(3):533–42.
4. Wetherell JL, Afari N, Rutledge T, et al. A randomized controlled trial of acceptance and commitment therapy and cognitive-behavioural therapy for chronic pain. Pain. 2011;152(9):2098–107.
5. Turk DC, Meichenbaum D, Genest M. Pain and behavioral medicine: a cognitive-behavioral perspective. New York: Guilford Press; 1983.
6. Halifax J. A heuristic model of enactive compassion. Curr Opin Support Palliat Care. 2012;6(2):228–35.
7. Solomon S, Greenberg J, Pyszczynski T. A terror management theory of social behavior: the psychological functions of self-esteem and cultural worldviews. Adv Exp Soc Psychol. 1991;24:93–159. https://doi.org/10.1016/S0065-2601(08)60328-7.
8. Ardnt J, Vess M, Cox C, Goldenberg J, Lagle S. The psychological effect of thoughts of personal mortality on cardiac risk assessment. Med Decis Mak. 2009;29(2):175–81.
9. Solomon S. The effects of mortality salience and neuroticism on medical students' treatment preferences for patients with terminal illnesses. Unpublished pilot data. Skidmore College; 1999.
10. Gilpin R. The use of Theravāda Buddhist practices and perspectives in mindfulness-based cognitive therapy. Contemporary Buddhism. 2008;9(2):227–51. https://doi.org/10.1080/14639940802556560.
11. Davidson RJ, Kaszniak AW. Conceptual and methodological issues in research on mindfulness and meditation. Am Psychol. 2015;70(7):581–92. https://doi.org/10.1037/a0039512.

Chapter 9
Class 7: Mindful Congruent Practice in Clerkship and Beyond

Tom A. Hutchinson

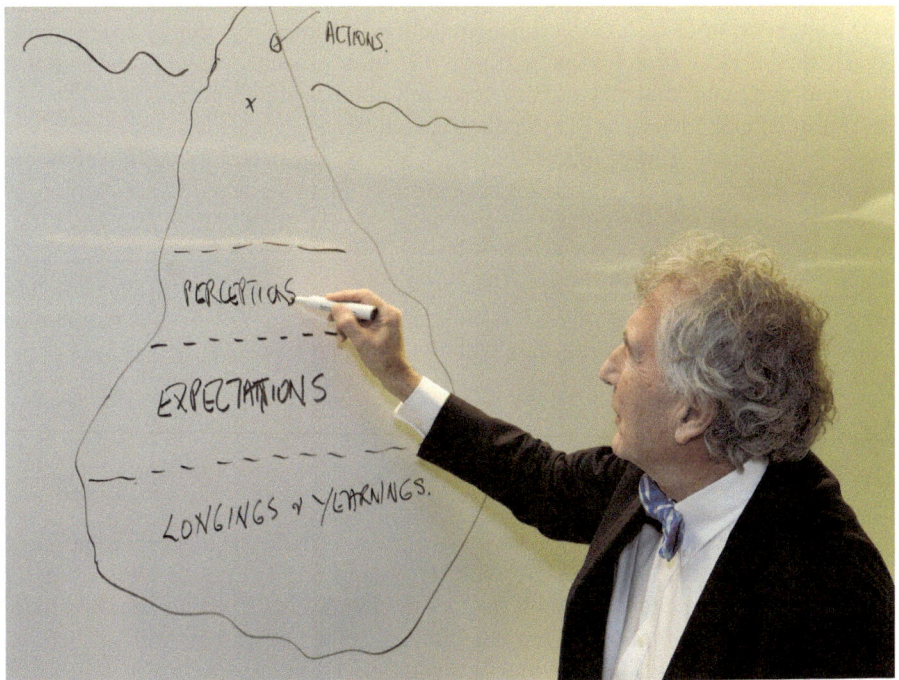

Fig. 9.1 Instructor drawing the iceberg metaphor

Overview

The purpose of this class is to complete the course so that students leave with a sense of energy and purpose to apply what they have learned in their upcoming clerkship. The class has three main phases: (1) an introductory phase where students

© Springer Nature Switzerland AG 2020   101
S. Liben, T. A. Hutchinson, *MD Aware*,
https://doi.org/10.1007/978-3-030-22430-1_9

are reminded to acknowledge their experience so far, (2) a deeply reflective part where we use the iceberg metaphor (Fig. 9.1) to help students examine their current internal response to clerkship, and (3) a completion ceremony.

This is an important transition point for the students but also for the teacher. It is likely that the teacher will have gotten to know and to like most if not all of the students in the class. You will probably sense that some of them have contributed a lot and have been deeply engaged. Consciously attempt to let go of any resentments against uncooperative students and do not make any last-minute attempts to reach students who may be on (or perhaps over) the fence.

The other possible tendency that you may need to be aware of is a desire to get this class and the course over as expeditiously as possible. This may be the case particularly in the unlikely event that the course has not gone well, but the tendency may be there regardless of how the course has worked. You have taught six classes in consecutive weeks, and it is a normal human tendency to be somewhat fatigued and to want to be finished. However, this is not the time to relax in your intention, to take it easy, or to rush to get finished. Remind yourself that this is a very important class, at least as important as those that have preceded it, and you owe it to yourself and to the students to give it your full mindful attention. There will be time to reflect and take it easy when the class is complete.

Having said all of this, the last class can also be a satisfactory culmination, and even celebration, of your time with this unique group of students. The iceberg metaphor is a perfect way to capture internal experience during points of important transition such as this, and it completes in a very powerful way what you have already taught students of the Satir material, particularly the stances. The completion ritual can be a perfect rounding off of this class and the course. Enjoy your moment-to-moment experience in the last class with this group of students!

1. Seated Guided Awareness Practice

We start the class with a guided awareness practice (GAP) that is, as far as possible, identical to that with which we began the course in Class 1 (Chap. 3). We do not tell the students of this intention, but if the first class began with paying attention to the left big toe, this meditation begins and continues in the same way.

This repetition of the GAP with which you began the course is relatively straightforward. Of course it may not be identical word for word, and you should not concern yourself about this. It needs to be similar enough so that some students have a sense of déjà vu and of the elapse of time and experience since the first class. The debrief should be fairly open-ended, but you should express particular interest in comments that indicate this reflective experience. If such comments do not come up, you might ask, "Did someone notice that this guided awareness practice was similar to the one with which we opened the first class?" as a way of stimulating discussion. Assuming students notice the similarity, they may describe how it was easier this time, or some students may say it was more difficult. You should let students know that both experiences are perfectly valid and even expected in the ups and downs of any experience of meditation.

2. "What Has Come Up Since Class 6 (Responding to Suffering)?"

We conduct this reflection by putting students in dyads. They pick an A and a B. Each of them is asked to take a moment to reflect on what they remember from the last class and any questions or issues it has raised in their minds. The interaction begins with A speaking and B listening for a timed 3 minutes. We then switch with B speaking and A listening for a further 3 minutes. The interaction is completed by giving the dyad 3 minutes to discuss between them what came up. You then open the floor to a large group discussion.

It is important to give students the opportunity to comment on the previous class. In some ways "Responding to Suffering" is the center of this course, and we want students to understand this by the way we deal with their reflections on Class 6 (Chap. 8). If you can, you should relate their comments to other classes in the course, to skills that they have learned, and to what is about to come up in Class 7.

3. The Iceberg Metaphor

This is the core of this class, a major transition point in the course, and a final opportunity for the group to feel a sense of shared internal experience as they contemplate clerkship. By this point in the course, students have come to know each other in ways that they had not previously experienced. So, this exercise aims to achieve two objectives: (1) to help students learn more about their own internal experience and (2) to realize how other students in the group share many similar longings, expectations, perceptions, feelings, and stances. Students find this enlightening, surprising, and often reassuring. They are not alone. This course is both an individual and a group experience, and this combined effect of the course is consolidated in this final major exercise.

In order to be familiar with the iceberg metaphor, you will need to read further on the topic in the works of Virginia Satir [1]. You will also need to practice going through your own iceberg with a colleague or colleagues. The distinctions between longings, expectations, and perceptions can be fairly subtle, and you will need the opportunity to explore these distinctions in some depth before presenting them to students. You will also need to be willing to take some risk of self-exposure to do an effective job of presenting your iceberg to the class. The temptation may be to pick

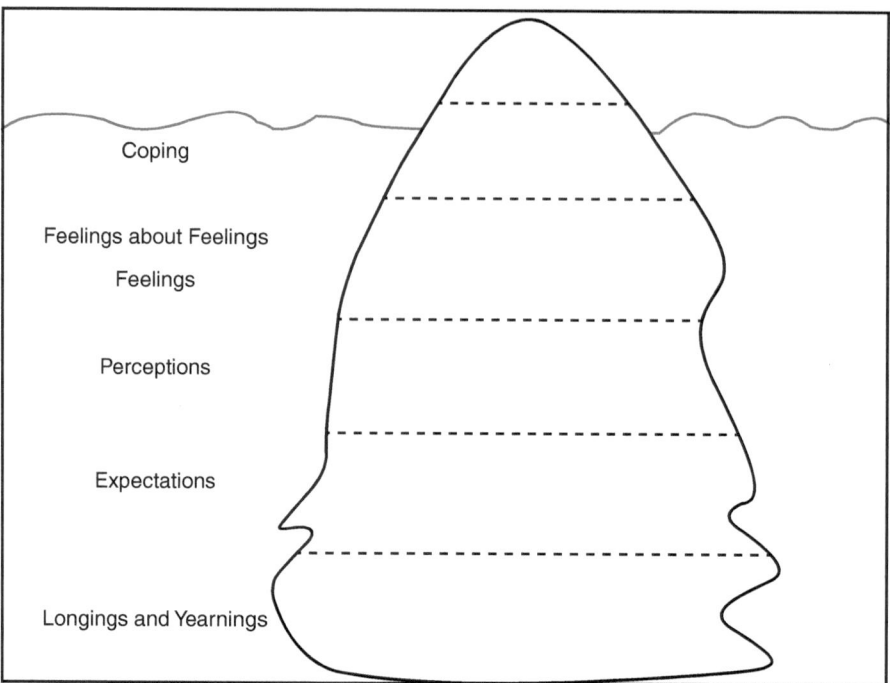

Fig. 9.2 Iceberg metaphor. (Recreated with permission from Satir et al. [1])

something safe. We would advise you to avoid this tendency and to pick an experience that is fresh for you and carries a sufficient emotional charge to ensure that you are fully engaged in your presentation.

We begin by reminding students briefly of the communication stances and point out that these are often just below our normal level of awareness. If this level of awareness is pictured as a water level, there is a lot more going on under the water – our personal iceberg. We draw a picture of the iceberg with the different levels (Fig. 9.2) and lead the students through our personal iceberg in relation to a past or future challenging personal transition (something major – e.g., a change in geographic location, a change in our job, expecting a child). We begin our personal iceberg at the bottom, the level of longings and yearnings.

- Longings and yearnings: We point out that these are very powerful but sometimes difficult to tap. We may even have learned to suppress our own longings, but they are there. Many of these are fairly generic such as a yearning to be loved, to be appreciated, to love, and to be truly happy. However, there may be an individual flavor to them. Describe as best as you can your personal longings in relation to the transition you have identified. One test of whether you have gotten in touch with your own longings is that the experience should be both energizing and somewhat embarrassing.

- Expectations: Expectations can be concretized longings ("This is how I expect you to love me.") or your sense of how things will be based on past experience ("I expect this will not work."). A good guide to expectations is that they will often include or imply the word "should" as in "You should express your love this way" or "He should agree with me."
- Perceptions: Perceptions are the meanings we give to what we are experiencing. So when looking at a future transition, my perception might be that this will be an adventure, a big mistake, or a painful experience.
- Feelings: We will have feelings triggered by our longings, expectations, and perceptions. These may be feelings of excitement, fear, anxiety, shame, and so on. Often these may be multiple, and we may have different conflicting feelings at the same time. A word of caution: statements such as "I feel that ..." are not feelings but actually perceptions or expectations. It may take a moment of focused attention to identify your feelings.
- Feelings about feelings: We have feelings about our feelings. For instance, if I feel angry, I may have a fear of that feeling. On the other hand, if I feel joyful, I may feel guilty about feeling joyful. It is often our feelings about our feelings that trigger our communication stance.
- Coping: These are the communication stances that we have previously described: placating, blaming, super-reasonable, and distracting.

After completing our own iceberg, we hand out the iceberg sheets (Appendix C) for students to complete their own icebergs as they contemplate clerkship. We take students through each stage starting with longings and yearnings. When you ask the students to do their own iceberg, stress that this is a metaphor. It is not right or wrong but a way that we have found useful in helping students explore their own psyches in more depth. Do not break students into dyads at this point or let them know that they will be asked to share their iceberg with another student. We would prefer that students first attempt to get as good a sense of their personal iceberg as possible.

When everyone has completed the iceberg sheet, we divide the class into dyads and ask them to share as much as possible of their personal icebergs with each other. Do not stress that they should only share what they are comfortable with – they will do this anyway. If students ask, you can confirm that they do not have to share more than they are willing to. When all dyads have completed their conversations, we open it up for general discussion.

Students will normally find this exercise insightful and stimulating. They may share how surprised they are at either the similarities or differences in their respective icebergs. If they have difficulty identifying their stance, a clue may be as follows: If expectations are the most easily identified part of their iceberg, they are likely in a blaming stance; if perceptions are easier, they may be in a super-reasonable stance; if feelings are easiest to be aware of, they may be in a placating stance; if none of the iceberg is easy to bring to awareness, they may be in a distracting stance. Students who are easily aware of all parts of their iceberg, including longings, may be congruent.

In the general discussion, you want to give students the opportunity to learn from what happened in other dyads – difficulties, insights, and questions that they have are all good bases for further discussion. As far as possible you want to stay with students' experience of the exercise rather than get diverted into analytical discussions. Do not encourage discussion of whether the iceberg is a good metaphor or how it relates to other ways of viewing the psyche. You might say that these are reasonable thoughts or questions but issues they may want to explore on their own outside the class or in another context. You would like to end the discussion leaving each student with a sense of their personal iceberg as it relates to clerkship and how that fits (probably very well) with what other students in the class are experiencing.

4. "Fire" by Judy Brown

Read the poem (Appendix D) slowly, and if you are comfortable with doing so, read it again. Ask students how they feel the poem relates to the previous iceberg exercise. This is an opportunity to allow students to reflect on what they have experienced in the iceberg exercise and to deepen that reflection. The issue of longings and expectations should come up as should the need for space between expectations. Some students may see logs as expectations and fire as longings, and this suggests that too many expectations (logs) may dampen the fire of longing. You should allow students to raise these issues, but even if they are not raised, do not be tempted to explain what the poem means to you. You will not take the students' understanding further than they can go spontaneously, and the poem may stay with them as a mystery that gets clarified long after the course is complete.

5. The Four Levels of Knowing

There are four levels of knowing:

1. Not knowing
2. Knowing
3. Realizing
4. Actualizing

Point out that we may know many things without fully realizing what they mean or actualizing their power in our lives. A good example is that we all know life is lived in the present moment. When else could it be lived? But we usually don't realize what it would mean to live fully in the present; in fact, we spend most of our time in our minds living in the past or the future. Actualizing would be fully experiencing what it is like to live fully in the present moment. In explaining these distinctions, a colleague finds the following example very helpful:

- *Not knowing*: The child less than age 5 does not even know what death is/means.
- *Knowing*: From ages 5–10, the child learns what death is as a concept and can explain it to others, including that it will happen to them one day.
- *Realizing*: An event happens that suddenly makes the child realize, in a moment, that he/she too will really die – this realization comes and goes from awareness.
- *Actualizing*: Living with the knowledge that we will each die, integrated into our thoughts and actions.

It may also be useful to give an example from your own life about a personal experience of realizing and actualizing. Avoid making this part of the class overly didactic. Ask the students to give examples from their own lives and use their answers as a basis for clarification. If they come up with explanations, ask, for example, to illustrate what they mean. Depending on how the discussion goes, you might want to ask them how this course fits into the distinctions they have made. Rather than leaving them with answers, you would like to leave them with ongoing personal questions about these distinctions. We finish this step by distributing "Tips for Mindful Practices" (Appendix E), which provides guidance for bringing awareness to their daily activities.

6. Discuss the Essay Assignment

We point out that the essay is a way of stimulating them to reflect on the class and clarifying for themselves what they found helpful and what they want to use as they move forward. There are two parts:

- In 500 words (minimum), describe your experience of participating in the course.
- In 750 words (minimum), outline which (and why) specific class themes and exercises may be particularly helpful in your future clinical practice.

Recapitulate for the students that the themes of the classes are as follows: Class 1, Attention and Awareness; Class 2, Congruent Communication; Class 3, Awareness and Decision-Making; Class 4, Clinical Congruence; Class 5, Building Resilience; Class 6, Responding to Suffering; and Class 7, Mindful Congruent Practice in Clerkship and Beyond.

The main exercises are GAP (Guided Awareness Practice), dyad discussions, large group discussions, viewing videos, acting out stances, role plays, and narrative exercises.

Some students may see the essay as another onerous job to do. Do not take on that point of view or be apologetic. Make a strong point that you will read every essay with your full attention and give them written feedback.

7. Closing Exercise

Before you begin the closing exercise, take a breath, deliberately slow down, and focus. Remind yourself that this is an opportunity to complete the course in a mindful and powerful way. Then take a few moments to explain to students what will occur. Request students stand in a cirlce. Stress the need for mindful pacing and attention.

Explain that this is a ritual to complete the class. In all rituals there needs to be a certain pace (relatively slow) and a focused attention to what is unfolding. You will hand around a pen in the order in which students are ready to speak. When they receive the pen, students should hold it for a moment and allow themselves to speak one word that expresses what they are left with in the present moment as the course completes. When they are finished, they hold the pen until the next student indicates they want to speak. The first student walks to give the pen to the next student and walks back. The student who intends to speak should wait until the circle is reformed.

You begin the exercise by holding up the pen and asking for the first student volunteer. There may be a delay, which is okay, and you will need to be present and accepting of your own anxiety if that arises. When the first student raises his/her hand, walk deliberately across the room, hand the pen, walk back to your spot, and nod to the student to speak. Behave as you want other students to do when they hand the pen. Be prepared to step in and redirect or slow things down if you feel things are going too quickly or otherwise becoming derailed. It will usually not take much to keep things on track. At some point all the students will have spoken, or some students will not have spoken, and there may be no more requests for the pen. Give a few moments to be sure (longer than feels completely comfortable), and if there are still no volunteers, take the pen yourself and mindfully allow the word that expresses what you are left with to emerge and be spoken. Declare the course complete!

See Table 9.1, Teaching template for Class 7.

Table 9.1 Teaching template. Class 7: Mindful Congruent Practice in Clerkship and Beyond

Core concepts	Materials	Time
Iceberg metaphor Difference between knowing and actualizing	Iceberg sheets and pens Poem "Fire" Tips for Mindful Practices printouts Essay requirements Markers for whiteboard	Minutes
1. **Seated Guided Awareness Practice (No Start Time)** "Bringing your attention to the sensation of your left foot as it makes contact with the ground…" – Should be identical to the very first class, *but* just start the exercise without telling them that (they will need to "catch on") Debrief awareness exercise and compare with 7 weeks ago		10
2. **"What Has Come Up Since Class 6 (Responding to Suffering)**?" A-B dyad discussion followed by large group reflection		15
3. **The Iceberg Metaphor** Start with reminding them of the stances, and point out that these stances are just below the waterline of our actions Draw an iceberg on the board with the water level indicated at the top just above coping stances but no other divisions marked in Mark in the divisions, and name the sections as you introduce them, starting at the bottom (yearnings)		5
Take them through the iceberg using yourself as an example, starting at longings and yearnings		10

Hand out iceberg sheets, and ask them to complete for themselves as they contemplate clerkship – take them through it step by step starting with longings
When complete break into dyads, and give 5 minutes each to discuss what came up. Which stances?
Large group discussion:
  If they have difficulty identifying their stance, a clue might be the part of the iceberg they are most aware of (expectations, blaming; feelings, placating; perceptions, super-reasonable; nothing, distracting)
  The key to congruence is bringing presence to deeper longings
		25

4. **"Fire" by Judy Brown** Read poem twice and discuss in the group Group should bring up connections to the iceberg and longings		10
5. **The Four Levels of Knowing** Write them on the whiteboard: (1) not knowing, (2) knowing, (3) realizing, (4) actualizing Distribute "Tips for Mindful Practices" printouts		10

6. **Discuss the Essay Assignment**
Explain intention: To help them clarify for themselves what they have learned that might be useful to them, particularly in their clinical work
Reflecting back on the MMP course write an essay to respond to these two topics:
  Minimum of 500 words: Describe your experience participating in the MMP course
  Minimum of 750 words: Outline which (and why) specific class themes and exercises may be particularly helpful or unhelpful in your future clinical practice
		10

(continued)

Table 9.1 (continued)

7. **Closing Exercise** Explain that this is a ceremony, or ritual, and needs to be carried out with a certain slowness and presence We will ask each student to say a word that expresses what they are left with at the end of this course Hand around a pen starting with the first person who volunteers, says a word, and then hands on the pen to the next volunteer Proceed until all of the students who want to have taken a turn Finish with a word from the leader(s) Declare the class complete	10

Reference

1. Satir V, Banmen J, Gerber J, Gomori M. The transformation process. In: The Satir model: family therapy and beyond. Palo Alto: Science and Behavior Books; 1991. p. 147–74.

Chapter 10
Live and In Person: One Class from Moment to Moment

Tom A. Hutchinson

This is based on an audio recording of Class 6 (Chap. 8): Responding to Suffering, taught by coauthor TAH on February 15, 2019.

1. G.A.P

Teacher: Get comfortable. Arms, legs not crossed, sit relatively straight, noticing your feet on the ground, see if you can just notice your breathing.

Noticing the in breath and the out breath.

As thoughts arise, your attention is taken elsewhere, something other than the breath, just allowing that to be, and then bringing your attention back gently, resting on your breath.

Like somebody sitting on the side of a stream, thoughts and feelings are drifting by. No need to go with them. Just sitting on the side of the stream. Just paying attention to your breathing.

Now, allowing your attention to expand to the sounds in the room.

See if you just can hear the sounds, not following the meaning that you would give to those sounds.

Nothing to do, nowhere to go.

Just noticing yourself sitting here, breathing and hearing sounds.

Sitting, noticing, breathing, listening to sounds.

As you are ready, in your own time, bringing your attention gently back to the room. If your eyes have been closed, allow them to open.

What did you notice?

Student: I had a whole lot of emotions and thoughts, a million things that I probably thought about, and it went away. Then that thing and that went away. I just felt like a series of thoughts coming. I could not stop them from coming.

S. Liben, T. A. Hutchinson, *MD Aware*,
https://doi.org/10.1007/978-3-030-22430-1_10

Teacher: Which is fine. And that's one of the things you notice in meditation. Feelings and thoughts arise and they disappear. Arise and disappear and that's fine. Anything else you've noticed?

Student: I am usually able to clear my mind. Today I wasn't. I am not sure why.

Teacher: Sometimes it's impossible to know why. There is a whole climate or a whole weather internally that we are not really aware of, and sometimes we can easily focus, and sometimes we can't. So it's OK. Just be aware of that.

2. Pain and Suffering

Teacher: Today the class is about suffering. First of all, I would like to hear from you some of your ideas about what is suffering. The word "patient" has the same origin as the word "to suffer." So, what is suffering?

Student: It sort of binds people together, something very human, that we all know, that we all share, and that often brings people together.

Teacher: Very good. It's interesting. It can bring people together, and we'll talk about it later, or it can pull people apart. Other thoughts about what is suffering?

Student: Are you talking about suffering in the context of health?

Teacher: Not necessarily, suffering in general, but if you want to give me something in the context of health, that's fine too.

Student: I guess it's something I don't like to think about. I know it's something we all share, and it's part of human life, but I'd like to put it aside.

Teacher: Very important. So whatever suffering means, we are not so keen to get into it. And we mostly would like to avoid it.

Student: There is suffering with the patients in the hospitals. Emotional suffering. It can totally drain someone.

Teacher: Yes, absolutely. Other thoughts about suffering?

Student: It can be very much determined by culture and society. One thing I am thinking about is the developing world. A common thought about the developing world is that there must be suffering all the time, as they don't have all the things they need. But when you go to the developing world, it's just suffering on a different level that you realize is not more or less relevant than it is here. There are different attributes and different causes. Another thing that made me think about cultural differences is pain management and how we really want to remove pain, because I guess pain and suffering go hand in hand, and in the West we tend to really want to control pain and alleviate it. Someone told me that in Germany, they try to prescribe less pain medication and try to have more of a focus on how pain is part of the healing process. Sort of a cultural thing, that pain is there for a reason and something I have to go through, and so there is less focus on trying to get rid of the physical pain. These are two examples that I thought will help on how society and culture really shape the perception of suffering.

Teacher: Very good. The other interesting relationship is pain and suffering. My question would be: Is there a situation where there is pain maybe even severe pain, but none or little suffering?

Student: Childbirth.

Teacher: Perfect example. Why would pain not be associated with suffering in that situation?

Student: It is the end goal. It's a small fraction. Negligible.

Teacher: Very good. Other thoughts?

Student: Maybe because there is pain from gaining rather than the pain from dying which is losing…

Teacher: It's very good. I'm going to come back to your point.

Student: It's also short term. You know that it's going to end, and at some point, you are going to be OK versus some people at the hospital, for instance. They don't know how long they will have this pain that they are struggling with. So, if you know that it is going to end at some point and you are going to be OK…

Teacher: It's very good. Those three points relate to something that is probably essential about suffering. The fact that in childbirth, it's only a small part of it, that most of it is good, and X's point that actually it means something good, as opposed to dying, and the other part is that if you have pain and you are not sure when it will end that's a different thing than knowing that this is going to end.

Student: It's like pain with purpose.

Teacher: Exactly. In the 1980's Eric Cassell published a paper, a very seminal paper, in the NEJM and subsequently wrote a book called *The Nature of Suffering and the Goals of Medicine*. And what he said is very simple. Suffering occurs when there is a threat to your intactness as a person. That will explain why, for instance, if you give birth to a child, it's actually not the same threat to your sense of intactness as a person; it's more like growth. If the same symptom is associated with an onset of a serious disease, or dying, or you never know when it's going to finish, that does affect your whole sense of life. "How am I going to live with this, what it's going to be like, if this doesn't finish, how will I be who I want to be?" That's the crucial aspect of suffering. For instance, I could develop a mild pain in my knee, which to you or even to my doctor would be: "What's the big deal?" Maybe that pain in my knee means to me that I am not going to be able to do something that I really love to do, like play tennis. If this is going to end my tennis game, I could be really suffering. I would say most patients who come to the hospital are suffering in exactly that way. They are thinking "What does this mean?" "Is there going to be a change in who I am?" That is suffering. Thoughts about that?

Student: I think that in a pediatric setting, there is often pain without suffering perhaps because of naivety which adds a negative connotation, but I mean it positively here. And also there is hope all the time because they always think it's going to end because why wouldn't it, and they do not have all of the baggage from a lifetime of experience. So I think especially in a pediatric setting, especially pediatric oncology, it's always "Well, that must be so hard," but I have a friend who is a nurse in pediatric oncology, and it is the best place to be. Adult oncology suffering, there is going to be no end, it's really disrupting my person. Pediatric oncology way brighter, way more hope and joy in the hospital.

Teacher: So you are saying that part of what we learn as we grow and mature is learning how to suffer more severely.

Student: I think it's not a conscious learning.

Teacher: It's not an intention.

Student: But unconsciously we just contribute and build up and build up in our psyche until….

Teacher: And that could be why Kabat-Zinn's work with chronic pain was effective. Because I think what he was trying to do is to get people more in the moment versus all of these future projections that threaten them.

Student: Who was the person?

Teacher: Jon Kabat-Zinn, who is the person who really has promoted and popularized mindfulness at the University of Massachusetts in the last 40 years. He started with people with chronic pain. I don't think he was changing the physical pain, but I think he was doing a lot for their suffering.

3. Helpful Versus Unhelpful Responses to Suffering

Teacher: One of your jobs, I would say your main job, is to relate to people who are suffering in a helpful way, and a lot of patients are suffering severely.

We are going to divide you into groups. Now, individually think of a time when you were suffering, and think of the people that you were relating to at that time. How did it work? It does not have to be medical. On this side, I would like you to think of ways of relating to your suffering that were not helpful. Make a list. On this side, think of ways that people related to you that were helpful. Go ahead. I will give you a few minutes, and then we will see what you think.

Students are talking in groups.

Teacher: OK. You may still stay in groups. We are going to start at this side. Give me one thing that you came up with that was helpful for your suffering.

Student: First thing we have is sharing familiar experiences.

Teacher: So, sharing. What exactly do you mean by "sharing a familiar experience"? So you are suffering. What is the other person doing that is helping?

Student: It's related to empathy. When somebody shares a similar situation and then you see that they got out of it.

Teacher: OK. They are sharing with you. I had a situation like that. Very good. Give me a helpful one here.

Student: It's being part of a community that is going through things together.

Teacher: Which is kind of related in some ways to the first one. You can see why community would be important to the main issue of suffering. You fear the loss of identity. "Who am I?" If there are other people around you who are supporting your identity, that's what community does, but also having the same thing, very helpful.

Give me an unhelpful thing.

Student: Just in contrast to the same thing that was said if they try to make it about them, when they do make it about them by sharing something, that probably is not good.

Teacher: It's very good. So, we could put "sharing" here too. But it's very true. If I am suffering and you say I know exactly how that feels, and …

Another unhelpful one here.

Student: Problem-solving instead of supporting.

Teacher: Very good. Something that we all tend to move to pretty quickly. Right? If you are suffering and you have a pain in your knee, the first thing I might do is "Oh, take some Tylenol." Is it all bad? No. But certainly it can be a problem. Because you are not really hearing me.

Give me a helpful one.

Student: I would just counter that by saying problem-solving. Because if we have shared enough and people have listened and then somebody can become a little more pragmatic and help you see the light at the end, help with coping.

Teacher: Absolutely. A lot of what medicine is about is exactly that. You are suffering because you have pain, but I can take away the pain, or we can fix the problem that is causing the pain. Very helpful.

Give me another helpful one.

Student: Someone who is really listening to you and not always saying "Oh, it happened to me too." "Oh, I had worse than that."

Teacher: Yes. Really listening is key.

An unhelpful one.

Student: They try to minimize what we are going through. It's not a big deal.

Teacher: Oh, it's not so serious. Other people had worse things. Minimize. There is no question that when you are suffering, the last thing you want is it minimized.

Another unhelpful one.

Student: When they make themselves feel better because they say they feel so bad about your situation. Like "I am so sad that you are sad." It's about making them feel better.

Teacher: So, focus on themselves and they feel better. OK. Can you give to me a helpful one?

Student: Sharing coping techniques, joining you to help you cope.

Teacher: Coping techniques. OK.

Another helpful one.

Student: People checking in. Saying that they care.

Teacher: Yes, so they don't just forget about it, they don't stop calling. "How is that going?" It's really important. Follow up. Checking in.

Give me an unhelpful one.

Student: When people try to touch us, something like a forced hug.

Teacher: Very good.

Another unhelpful one.

Student: When you feel the person is not genuine.

Teacher: They are really not taking in what you are saying. Not genuine.

Student: False reassurance.

Teacher: A helpful one.

Student: Giving hope that it's going to pass.

Teacher: Hope. OK.

Another helpful one.

Student: Validation for suffering.

Teacher: Validation, very important. Validation is key and that's one of the things we can do in medicine, right? People are suffering and maybe nobody is really getting them. They need to hear that it is not surprising that you are suffering in this case. This is a difficult thing.

An unhelpful one.

Student: Avoidance, they try to avoid it.

Teacher: Avoiding it in yourself but we avoid it in other people who are suffering too. We just don't want to know about it.

Give me a last unhelpful one.

Student: I know that it is related to the avoidance one but denial.

Teacher: Absolutely. Denial. Is there any other burning helpful or unhelpful one that you think should be on the list?

Student: For helpful, physical contact, especially maybe in a person who is chronically in the hospital and avoided and never touched.

Teacher: Make some contact. Very good.

Any other ones?

Student: For helpful. Company is always nice.

Teacher: Company. And close to community, right? Just having people around. Doesn't have to be your community but just having people around.

Student: Criticism for unhelpful. "Well, you chose the wrong boyfriend."

Teacher: Yes, it's easy to do, right? "What do you expect?"

Any others that you think are burning?

Student: For unhelpful, I would put unhealthy coping techniques. Like I have friends who are just saying "Let's go drink." That's not really helpful. It makes me more depressed. Although it can be helpful.

Teacher: Yes. One of the things you will notice about these lists is that it is a very subtle thing. The same thing can be helpful or unhelpful. So the physical contact, problem-solving, and so on can be helpful or unhelpful. How do you think these lists relate to the Virginia Satir stances? See any relationship?

Student: I could think of some of them being placating.

Teacher: So which ones would you call placating?

Student: Problem-solving could be unhelpful.

Teacher: It could be placating, yes.

Student: Placating can be non-genuine.

Teacher: Yes.

Student: Like sharing your experiences with a person and overdoing it.

Teacher: So where would that be? It could be placating for sure.

Student: Problem-solving as computer brain.

Teacher: Problem-solving definitely could be computer brain. It does not have to be only that but it certainly could be. It could be "Here's your problem, here's what you should do about it."

Student: I would say criticism blaming.

Teacher: Yes, definitely. Any others?

Student: Minimizing.

Teacher: Minimizing would be what?

Student: Also blaming.

Teacher: Yes.

Student: I would put problem-solving in the helpful category as congruent.

Teacher: It could be congruent. The thing about it is if suffering is mostly about your loss of identity and fear of loss of identity, then what's crucial is how I relate to you. If I am relating genuinely to you, hearing what you are saying, and trying to put myself in your shoes but not thinking I am you, then I am congruent. If I am rushing to solve the problem because I can't bear to even think about this, that could be computer brain. So, certainly it could be congruent. Other thoughts about this?

Student: A lot of the things that are either helpful or unhelpful are more often unhelpful in the context of computer brain. For example, maybe problem-solving could be very helpful given the context of the patient and what they need, but then if actually you are not paying attention to how they are responding to what you are saying and doing, then it becomes unhelpful computer brain. The same with physical contact. You can say that could be very helpful for someone who seems that they want that, but if you are not paying attention to them, it could actually be the opposite because you are just assuming it could be helpful – computer brain like.

Teacher: Perfect. Absolutely true. Other thoughts about this?

Student: I could put avoidance in the helpful category actually. In the unhelpful category, I would say you are in the distracting stance; in the helpful category, I would say it's when you are in the congruent stance and you can see that a little bit of distraction is what is needed right now. Dwelling on things with the suffering is not what's needed but just getting out and forgetting about it.

Teacher. Very good. If you think about somebody you know who is suffering, you don't want to be always reminding them about the suffering. "How is that now?" "How is that now?" It just makes it worse, right? So there is a certain point when you need to stop talking about it and you need to know how to pick that up. And maybe do something which is distracting, because the other point about that is if this is about who you are and your sense of identity, to do something normal is very affirming to your sense of who you are. So if I am suffering and I am worried about the future, to go to a movie, if that's something we normally do, and I can enjoy that movie to some extent, that's a reaffirmation, I am still involved in life here. Very tricky. Other thoughts about this?

Student: I think that if you take any stance that is not congruent, it makes everything that you do go from helpful to unhelpful.

Teacher: I think that's a brilliant summary. I would say that's true. If I am blaming you, placating you, if I am being super reasonable, distracting, out of a lack of a sense of awareness either of you, or me or the context, I will probably not be very helpful. So it is more about how I am really relating to you than about the specific things that I do.

4. Awareness of Time Exercise

Teacher: I am going to do an exercise now. It's going to raise an issue that is very confronting. It's either very problematic or very helpful. Let's have some paper and I will tell you what to do.

Every student is taking one sheet of paper with the Goals and Dreams exercise.

Teacher: What I want you to do now is write down five goals or dreams that you have for your life right now. That's the start. Five things that you would love to see happening to you.

Students write.

Teacher: I want you to pair up and share your goals and dreams. If there is a goal or dream that you are too embarrassed about, don't share it. Don't cross it out, but don't share it.

Students talk.

Teacher: Ok. Let's bring that to a close. So, the bad news is that you have just been diagnosed with lung cancer. It can happen at any age. I had somebody to whom I gave a course like this who the following Monday was actually diagnosed with metastatic cancer. You have been diagnosed with lung cancer. This is a problematic cancer, it is metastatic, not curable, you are coughing a bit, but the expectation is that you will live about a year. So now, look at your goals and dreams, and see how they change if you have approximately a year to live. Go ahead.

Take a moment separately just to look at your goals and dreams and then discuss. You don't have to rewrite them, you can remove some, you can add some, but if you have all five new write all five.

Students write.

Teacher: You can share whenever you are ready.

Students talk.

Teacher: If you can bring that to a close. A little time has gone by. The cancer is progressing much more rapidly, as often happens. Now we are talking about weeks to months. You are sicker but not in terrible pain; they are controlling your pain well; you can walk around, but you are not well, and it looks like about a month. So, if it was a month, what would now be your goals and dreams? Go ahead. Do it separately first and then discuss.

Students write.

Teacher: When you are ready, you can discuss.

Students share in pairs.

Teacher: Bring that to a close. They were not wrong. Things are progressing rapidly. You are now in palliative care. You are in bed, not in pain, you are not delirious, but people think now it is a question of days. I have seen people exactly in that state, at your age, it is not impossible. What would now be your goals and dreams for whatever time is left? First of all write down and then discuss them. Go ahead.

Students write.

Teacher: When you are ready discuss. There is no rush.

Students discuss.

Teacher: You can bring that to a close.

Teacher: What did you notice in that process?

Student: The element of time was always the determinant of the goals. The less and less time I have, the more accessory stuff started to drop out, and it became more about family and friends. It was also hard.

Teacher: Hard, yes, definitely. Other people notice similar things or different things?

Student: When at first we did not have the sickness, we were OK; one of the things I had at med school, was like to be knowledgeable, be a good clerk, and then as soon as I had a year left, that disappeared. I don't know what that tells you about me but medicine was not there anymore. I think that this is because we are not yet doctors; if we were it would be maybe like do my work and help the people, like right now we are not really helping, so it is not really necessary to do that.

Teacher: Very good. Other things? What did you notice?

Student: I don't know if that's true. I understand the point of exercise. When you are facing your own mortality, you come to realize who your true self is. You start up with a list of 5 to 100, and then things that are less important are crossed out, and in the end, at your last breath, you have 1 last thing that you really care about. It's like an exercise that you do. You know you are not going to die tomorrow; all of us are not going to die tomorrow.

Student: God willing.

Teacher: You do not know that.

Student: I know there is a good chance I am not going to die tomorrow, but if you do this exercise every day and you just make ends meet tomorrow with people you need to make ends meet with, then you can live a happier life.

Teacher: It's a good point that you might want to make the amends now versus putting things off, and this should put you in touch with that.

Student: I think that in a way I disagree with the idea that you cross out things that aren't as important to you. Because a lot of things can be maybe the most important to you but you have to suppress them for the time that you have left. For example, having a family is by far the most important thing to me now, but if I have only 1 year left, it does not make sense for me to have a child, so it's hard because it's a mix of what is really important to you in the moment but also realizing your long-term goals are not possible anymore.

Student: I have somewhere like top goal to have children and grandchildren, but I would say that throughout my list, things like having a family is consistently on my list. Having a kid right away, if I have 1 year left. I could freeze my eggs if I have only a month. I would like to be survived by a child.

Teacher: Part of that is legacy. Very good.

Student: At first it was all good, I would like to do that, I would do that, and so on. After that, for 1 year, I would just travel, and I would enjoy how much time I have left, throw a huge party, and then for months, I would probably focus on family, and then for a few days, I would make sure that my parents know how amazing they were to me because when you realize that if tomorrow I die for whatever reason and they don't know what an amazing job they did, that would be so much harder for them. I just think they will blame themselves, not knowing that they were amazing, and it will be much harder on them. It's more for them than for me.

Teacher: It's very good. Other thoughts before we go to the next piece?

Student (addressing another student): I'll try to say it very quick. But your comment that we are not going to die tomorrow, I'm not trying to say something very negative against your comment, but just in general, I feel like that there is some sort of ageism there because I think that the likelihood that I die tomorrow is identical to my 85-year-old grandfather. Because something in the fact that you are going to die tomorrow is something that is going to be abrupt, it's going to be a trauma, and it's going to be a massive heart attack. Maybe he has risk factors and the percentages are changing, but the idea that we all have way more time, I don't think that there is a huge difference, maybe 1% to 10%; it's not like my grandfather has 95% more chance to die tomorrow, so I don't agree at all that we are not going to die tomorrow.

Student: Hopefully no one dies tomorrow!

Laughter…

Teacher: You can see what a scary thought that is. Because what does everybody do? They laugh. But not an unrealistic thought. I don't think.

Student: You mentioned that a person wants to have a happy family. As soon as I have 1 year left, I actually did not want to have kids. I want to somehow convey to my wife that what I would want for her is to find somebody else and have kids with them. And I really did want to avoid having kids with her so that she does not deal with a constant reminder that I am no longer there. That is a huge difference in that if I have the last year to live, I want my wife to understand the way I am going to die happy is somebody is going to take care of her and she can have a family with him.

5. Terror Management Theory and Mortality Salience

Teacher: Very interesting. So, you can see that this gets you in touch with something, looking at your values, what's really important, elements of the future, elements of generosity, and elements of relationship. There has been actually quite some work done, mostly by psychologists Solomon, Greenberg, and Pyszczynski, on what happens when you trigger someone's "mortality salience," their awareness of their own mortality. What they found was interesting and quite different to your experience. Here is what they found. The first experiment was with judges, and these judges were randomly assigned to answer a questionnaire that they thought had to do with their personalities and how did that relate to the judgments made. The judgment that they had to make was to set bond for a woman accused of prostitution. The bond was the amount that this woman had to pay to get out of jail until her trial. If she couldn't pay the bond, she had to stay in jail. One half of the judges received the usual questionnaire and they asked them the personality things. The other half of the judges received the same questionnaire but with two additional questions to trigger their mortality salience. One of the questions was "Please briefly describe the emotions that the thought of your own death arouses in you" and something else that triggered their mortality salience. They compared the bond set by the judges who didn't have their mortality salience triggered versus the others. The judges in the control group set the bond at $50.00. Fifty dollars this woman would pay to get out of jail. What do you think the judges who had their mortality salience triggered set the bond at?

A few students: Zero.

Teacher: Zero?

Student: Five hundred dollars.

Teacher: You know this study?

Student: Yes, I have seen this study before.

Teacher: Z is right. It is actually $450.00. So, in fact they multiplied by roughly ten times the bond that was set. Their explanation for that is interesting. First of all, our awareness of mortality is probably somewhere there in our subconscious all the time, and our first defense against it is simply to suppress it or deny it. That's why when you ask people if they are thinking about their mortality, most people will say "no, not really." They don't really think about it. That's level 1. Level 2 is what they call the distal defenses. What these researchers say is that mortality is the greatest possible threat to our sense of who we are. Tomorrow I could simply not be here. It is very bad for your self-esteem, and so what you want to do when your mortality comes to the surface is to defend your self-esteem in some way, and the way people do that is they become more attached to and more associated with groups they feel share their values and they distance themselves from people who have different values. So, the theory is that this woman who practices prostitution is definitely not part of the judges' group; she does not represent their values, so they are willing to be quite tough on her. The opposite would be true for someone who shared their values. These researchers have done all kinds of studies on this. They wrote books called *In the Wake of 9/11*, *The Psychology of Terror*, and *The Worm at the Core: On the Role of Death in Life*. One of their conclusions is, for instance, that the whole American reaction to 9/11 is a perfect example of terror management. You feel threatened, you associate more with other Americans, and you distance yourself much more definitely from Muslims, foreigners, anybody who is different. More American flags, less tolerance. They've done studies in medicine. They took a group of medical students, these were Christian medical students, and asked them to evaluate the risk of serious heart disease in a variety of patients with different symptoms. Some of these patients were Christians and some were Muslims. Before they had their mortality salience triggered, the students gave about the same risks to the two groups; they seemed to be judging the two groups very similarly. But when they triggered their mortality salience, the students were much more worried about the

Christian patients and put the risks for the Muslim patients much lower. First question for you: How do you think this could play out in medical practice?

Student: Sometimes you get more affected by people who share more values with you than by those you don't relate with. If, for example, there is a person coming who has drug problems, whose life is conflicted and can't do the job properly, I feel like well, I am not going to worry so much about him as I would for a mother with three children. I really want to help her. That is obviously not a conscious decision, but I can imagine that my subconscious is biased.

Teacher: Absolutely. And does this happen? A lot. Very easy to happen. Just to be clear. Medicine triggers our mortality salience all the time. You can't be in medical practice, go to a hospital without at some level your mortality salience being triggered. So, that's definitely one level. Other ways in which this might play out in medical practice?

Student: Across age groups. Thinking "Oh, why would I put her on a statin, she is 88, you know, she is at the end of her life?" Well, because it is still indicated and who is to say when her life ends. So it's a big common thing, and I really find myself doing that, and the more I think about it, it is healthy because definitely before med school, "Ah, well, that's OK they lived their whole life." Does that mean that I think a young life is worth more? That's not really fair. So, definitely across age groups, it is very easy to put more emphasis on the young than the old.

Teacher: Definitely. Other ways in which this may play out? So, it could play out with different cultures and different ages. Are there any cultural groups within medicine that you may feel associated with or not?

Student: We all have different backgrounds; just in this room, we have a variety of cultural backgrounds, social status, and, all that, schools. With the degree of empathy you feel for other people, it's true that if you are a single mom, you may feel more empathy for a single mom at the hospital. You might feel more inclined to give more of your service to that person than another person. But I just feel that everybody has that.

Teacher: You are right, it is there. You all have cultural differences, it's true. Do you realize that this class in medical school is also becoming part of a culture? You are sharing the culture of medicine. What other groups are in the hospital that are not part of that cultural group?

Student: Patients.

Teacher: So, it is very easy for this to trigger that kind of response which is "we are the healthy ones and they are the sick ones," so distancing yourselves from patients. Does that happen? I think so, very much. Just to give you a quick example. I hadn't realized how powerful this was for me. I had a nurse I knew very well, a very nice person. I had not seen her for a while. Then somebody said to me: "Did you hear that Mary has metastatic breast cancer?" I was in my 30s. I met Mary in the corridor of the Old Vic, and I could hardly talk to her. It shocked me. I lost the words. What was that? That was weird. What I think it was is that I had a model of the world which was that we doctors and nurses are on the good side of the medical divide, we are on the side to stay healthy, and those patients they are on the other side. And now Mary had broken that rule. She was now on the other side. That's the only explanation that I had. I do think it is a very powerful effect, and probably it does explain a lot of the tendency of doctors to distance themselves from that whole patient group. But, here's the question. That did not seem to be the same thing, or was it, that happened to you when your mortality salience was overtly triggered. What is the difference between what these researchers are talking about and what you have experienced? Any thoughts?

Student: Maybe because it seems to me that their mortality saliency was triggered and tested as to how it would affect their profession. The medical students did not have a test to look at how it affects ourselves and our goals.

Teacher: Yes, it could be part of it.

Student: We are not doctors yet.

Teacher: It could be part of it. It's not I think the answer but it could be part of it. Any other ideas?

Student: The difference is overt versus covert.

Teacher: Exactly. In all those tests, people did not even know that their mortality salience was being triggered. It happened surreptitiously. In your case, there is no question that your mortality was out there in the open and you were asked to face it. And I do believe that's the answer. And they have actually done some experiments showing that if you trigger awareness of mortality overtly, it does not have the same effect. For me the idea would be if you want to deal with this, the way to deal with it is to more consciously be aware of your own mortality, because the extent to which you are aware of your own vulnerability allows you more easily to take a larger view of the world and not go with your own cultural group vs another cultural group. There is a certain generosity there. The other part of this is how you empathize with another person. This has very much to do with first of all facing your own vulnerability. I can't even empathize with you and your vulnerability unless I am willing to look at my own vulnerability because that is the level that we share. So, part of being congruent and being empathetic, I think, is to be willing to face our vulnerability and mortality. Does that make sense?

Student: I don't know whether you can go to a hospital and see people dying all the time and being empathetic towards that, and think about your own mortality, and then do that every day for the rest of your life. I guess that would be very exhausting.

Teacher: It is certainly anxiety provoking. Where does this happen in the hospital?

Student: Palliative care.

Teacher: In my experience of palliative care, it was exactly that. In palliative care you cannot possibly be unaware of your own mortality and patients' mortality. You can't do the job. It's anxiety provoking, but it's certainly possible to do it day after day. In fact, it's very rewarding. So, it's a strange kind of effect. And I think in a palliative care unit, that's what you notice. I would say, no, it's not exhausting, it's actually energizing. It's anxiety provoking, but it's not depressing.

6. "Just Like Me" Guided Visualization Exercise

Teacher: We are going to do an exercise on the process of putting yourself in someone else's shoes, being in touch with your own vulnerability, and then connecting with them on their vulnerability. It's a meditation. Let me ask you to just get comfortable again. If you can bring your mind to a person that you are very close to that you really have a lot of affection, love for. Picture that person in front of you. Say to yourself internally the following kinds of words:

"This person has suffered, been in pain, been afraid, just like me."

"This person has worried about the future, probably is worrying about the future, just like me."

"This person longs to be free of suffering, pain and discomfort, and worry. Just like me."

"This person longs to be happy, healthy, and fulfilled. Just like me."

Allow that person to fade. Picture somebody that you are not so close to. It could be a friend. Somebody you know well but you don't have strong negative feelings or strong positive feelings about him/her. Just picture that person. Say to yourself internally the following kinds of words:

"This person has suffered, this person has been in pain, this person has worried, just like me."

"At times this person has been unhappy, not knowing what to do, just like me."

"This person longs to be free of suffering, pain, and discomfort, and worry. Just like me."

"This person longs to be happy, healthy, and satisfied. Just like me."

Allow that person to fade. Picture a person with whom you have some difficulty. This is not somebody that you have a huge difficulty with or has done something unforgivable in your mind. This is somebody with whom somehow you don't feel so happy, or feel somewhat negative about them, have some criticism of them, maybe you have a hard time seeing their point of view. Picture that person in front of you. Say to yourself words something like the following:

"This person has suffered, been in pain, and worried, just like me."

"This person has been unhappy, not knowing what to do at times, feeling lost perhaps. Just like me."

"This person longs to be free of suffering, and pain, and worry. Just like me."

"This person longs to be happy, fulfilled, and satisfied. Just like me."

Allow that person to fade.

Just take a minute or two noticing your breathing. As you are ready in your own time, just bring your attention back to the room. If your eyes have been closed, allow them to open. So, what did you notice in doing that exercise?

Student: In the last one you mentioned, someone less close, a little bit different than I thought, I had not been feeling particularly good about the person, overtly mad at them. I think it humanized that person to remind myself that they are more than just what's been going on between us.

Teacher: Very good. Exactly what it is meant to do. Other things you've noticed?

Student: It wasn't hard. I guess I saw where the exercise was going, and I was thinking there will be a difference in terms of how I felt or how much it takes to convince myself…I was surprised.

Teacher: Very good. Because I think that when you get below that surface of disapproval, there is a level at which you absolutely connect. And that's the kind of level you are looking for in any kind of helpful connections with a person, including patients. Correct?

Student: Yes.

Teacher: Yes, if you want a last comment.

Student: I thought of the last two people. It occurred to me that these last two people also feel fear, worry. And I realized that while I am going on with my day I say to myself "Oh that person just is, they don't feel the same thing that I am feeling. Woe is me, I have so many problems." They have this whole thing happening with them, but I don't realize what's going on.

Teacher: Excellent. Perfect way to finish. It was kind of a deep morning. Class is finished.

Chapter 11
Mindful Medical Practice and the Good Doctor

Stephen Liben

Not Knowing → Knowing → Realizing → Actualizing

Learning new facts is not the only, or even necessarily the most important, aspect of becoming a good doctor. In Class 7 (Chap. 9), a conceptual model of learning that begins from "not knowing" and progresses to "knowing," "realizing," and then "actualizing" is outlined as one way to explore this together with students. In the first 1.5 years of medical school, referred to as the "pre-clinical" years (also sardonically referred to as the pre-cynical years), attention is necessarily focused on having students progress from "not knowing" foundational concepts in physiology and pathophysiology to "knowing" and proving that they know by answering exam questions that test their factual cognitive understanding. Further medical education is then an ongoing process of learning how to apply what is known, that is, "the facts," to the complex needs of ill human beings. The Oxford Dictionary defines the word "clinical" as "relating to the observation and treatment of actual patients rather than theoretical or laboratory studies." To practice "clinical" medicine is therefore to acknowledge that knowing facts is not enough and that to help actual patients requires wisdom and judgment in how to best apply what is already known. One way to answer the question of what has worked well in medical education would be to look at what has stood the test of time, to look at the educational practices that have not changed. Medical education, even in this era of needing to prove the "value added" by each new proposed educational intervention, still explicitly recognizes that much of what needs to be learned cannot be taught by listening to lectures and by simply reading the medical literature. How do we know this? We know that learning by doing, by experiencing, is valued in medical education because medical school curriculums still consist of large periods of time where students work with more senior physicians (residents and attending staff) in a modern version of apprenticeship that is called clerkship. After almost 2 years of clerkship, the medical school graduate will be granted an MD degree but is still not ready for independent practice. A further multi-year postgraduate period of apprenticeship, called residency, is still required before the postgraduate is able to practice medicine independently. Apprenticeships are expensive to run, require limited expert human resources, are difficult to regulate, and are notoriously hard to standardize. If there was any other way to learn than by spending years in apprenticeship, it would almost certainly be cheaper, faster, and easier to replicate. If the clerkship and residency apprenticeship phases of undergraduate and postgraduate medical education could, for example, be replaced by online courses, they no doubt would be replaced faster than public phone booths are being replaced by cellphones. Then why is medical education still dependent on mentor-guided "learn as you do" apprenticeships, despite the obstacles and difficulties involved? We would say that within medicine there remains a recognition, not always made explicit, that there are clear limits to what can be learned in lecture halls and by reading and absorbing facts. Rather, to be an effective physician means to learn *experientially* that which cannot be learned any other way.

As Mindful Medical Practice (MMP) is very much focussed on the practical application of knowledge to individual patients, it is very much a "clinical" course that offers students the opportunity, in class, to realize the practical application (clinical relevance) of some of what they have learned. For example, students learn about the Satir stances and then get to both experience for themselves and practice how these stances are received in role plays. Teaching that aims to have students go from not knowing to knowing is an essential step that can be effectively done by activities that include memorizing and developing cognitive understanding of concepts, by listening to lectures and personal reading. On the other hand, moving from "knowing" a concept as simple as understanding the importance to patients of being listened to and heard, to "realizing" deeply how much being listened to matters, requires personal engagement with a felt-experience, a "realization." Creating the conditions for such moments of realization is intentionally how classes are structured. Most students who come to Class 6 (Chap. 8) would say that they already know the importance of listening, but do they realize just how important it truly is? If they don't realize the salience of listening to patients, then why would we, as medical educators, expect them to be able to actualize listening in day-to-day clinical encounters? In Class 6, students engage in a deep listening exercise that has them see and feel for themselves, to realize what it is to both listen deeply and be deeply listened to. This deep listening exercise cannot guarantee that each student will experience the importance of deep listening, but rather creates conditions where such realizations are more likely to occur. Once students have the realization experience themselves, their learning is further consolidated by their peers, who in the small group articulate what they have learned. Students experience a realization in an exercise and then hear similar realizations being articulated by their peers in group discussions. Such "realizations" are what MMP classes are designed to create, and in-class discussions then consolidate learning by giving students the vocabulary to describe their experience and to compare and validate what they have learned.

MMP classes then have two interrelated learning objectives. The first objective is to ensure that students go from "not knowing" to "knowing" the basic conceptual knowledge that each class is built upon. These are the kinds of conceptual under-standings that are listed in course objectives and are easily tested using multiple-choice questions (e.g., the definitions of concepts). The second critically important objective is to create moments of "realization" for students so they can experience, on a nonconceptual level, what these concepts might mean to them, to their patients, and to their colleagues. Moments of realization are created by in-class exercises that bring awareness of cognition (thinking) together with moment-to-moment physical sensations (sensing) and emotional reactions (feeling), as outlined in the Triangle of Attention (see Chap. 7, Class 5) that was conceptually used to under-stand the relationship between attention and awareness. While traditional educa-tion is focussed on what students think, the process of learning through realization incorporates what students feel both emotionally and physically. By bringing awareness to thoughts, feelings, and sensations, we posit that students will gain more than knowledge:

> Knowing is not enough; we must apply. Willing is not enough; we must do. – Johann Wolfgang von Goethe

To bring what is known and has been realized into day-to-day life is to actual-ize facts into wisdom. Actualizing what has been learned is not an event but is rather an ongoing unfolding iterative process. The limits of human capacities mean that we can know what to do and why, and we may have had multiple moments of realizing for ourselves, but that does not mean that we will never again go against our own better judgment. Even experienced physicians who know the importance of listening to patients may nonetheless find themselves interrupting them at times. We may have moved along the learning spectrum from not knowing to actualizing, but that does not eliminate the multifaceted personal, social, and environmental attributes that come together at times to overwhelm even the wisest physician who "knows better" but nonetheless acts unhelpfully. The MMP course creates an environment for students to experience for them-selves (within moments of "realizations") how they might best apply the medical facts they are learning to help patients. There are many accounts of physicians who find out "what really matters" in their careers and lives only when they them-selves are faced with their own terminal diagnosis, such as in the end of life writ-ings of the physician Roger C. Bone [1]. Our explicit objective is to offer students learning experiences (realizations) so that they do not need to wait for their own life-threatening diagnosis to better understand what really matters to themselves and to their patients.

What Parts of the Course Can I Change?

There will inevitably be pressures from medical schools to modify MMP so that it would be easier to administer, less labor intense, more uniform and standard-ized, and given over less time. We would say that before making any changes to the curriculum, careful thought should be given to understanding the impact of proposed changes on the learning objectives of the course. Once each element of why and how the course requires the time and human resources that it does is appreciated, then changes can be made to the curriculum that continue to fulfill its main objective, that is, to have students experience for themselves realizations that can lead to the actualization of medical knowledge into clinically relevant skills. The duration (120 minutes) of each class, the number of students per class, and the total duration of the course (number of classes over a set time period) are structured based in part on the outcomes of previous mindfulness-based interventions [2].

Why Is Each Class 90–120 Minutes Long?

Each of the seven small group classes requires between 90 and 120 minutes and includes contemplative-based practices that help create the realizations of the learning objectives for that class. The structure of each class is purposively designed to create a level of student attention that goes deeper within the first 30–45 minutes of each class. Class time is oriented to the development of an ongoing dynamic small group relationship. Each class has some element of repetition, of novelty, of unexpected surprises, of concrete clinical examples, and of emotional intensity that is curated to unfold in an unhurried process. We have also purposively spaced and varied class activities to refresh students' attention by creating a change in pace about every 10–20 minutes. Exercises are spaced and timed so that sitting and talking alternate with moving, standing, and being silent. Every 20–40 minutes, students are asked to do something different that includes deliberately having them physically move or not move; think about what they are thinking, feeling, or sensing; and participate on their own, in dyads, or in large group work. We find that the 90–120 minutes of class time passes quickly for us as teachers, and that the majority of students are actively engaged for the entire class. We purposively do not provide a "break" during the 90–120 minutes, as we feel that energy and focus would be lost and would have to be regathered afterwards. If students absolutely need to leave during the class, they can simply leave and reenter as in any adult education course. MMP teachers gain student trust and respect over time, both within and between classes, as students see for themselves that the goal of MMP teachers is to have them learn essential clinical skills (see section on "safe-enough space" later in this chapter). What doctors need to know, in terms of essential cognitive concepts such as the pathophysiological mechanisms of disease, can be learned in large group lectures, in online courses, and through self-study. On the other hand, how to be with and assist sick patients requires more than listing cognitive facts and includes relational skills and self-awareness that are best learned via personal experience. Guiding students to experientially realize these non-purely cognitive skills requires the kind student-teacher relationship that the 90–120-minute MMP class, which includes small group peer-to-peer learning, cultivates.

Why Not Make the "Small" Groups Larger?

Group classes that are too large risk students feeling "unseen" and not known by the teacher, and we have found that with more than about 25 students it is more challenging to get to know each student. With a class that has less than about eight students, there is a risk of a lack of heterogeneity of student experiences to share and work with. With too small a group, there is also the risk that any particular student may feel too much attention focused on them personally and the intensity of interactions can at times be excessive for both student and teacher. We have found that groups of 15–25 students work best, and we now aim for 20 students per small group as our ideal number.

Why Run MMP Over 7 Consecutive Weeks?

A course duration of 7 weeks allows time for questions to come up and for learning to be reinforced by personal experiences between classes. While it may be possible to affect learning in less time than 7 weeks, it is harder to do so in a way that would work for the range of learning styles and capacities of an entire class of medical students. On any particular day, some students will be preoccupied with unavoidable life crises or their own physical or psychological obstacles that make learning less likely. Because our intention is to affect long-term changes in attitudes (e.g., seeing the lack of benefit of maintaining a blaming stance with patients) and in attentional skills (e.g., in bringing attention back to the patient during deep listening), there needs to be repetition of practice. Additionally, as classes progress from the first to the seventh class, the developed group dynamic and comfort that has been built up within the first classes on attention and communication are then used to help students grapple with the more demanding themes of human suffering and mortality in later classes.

"Safe Space" Versus "Safe-Enough Space"

The progression of what is being asked of students over time allows for the group dynamic to develop with enough trust in each other and in group process to facilitate the more emotionally demanding experiences of Classes 5, 6, and 7 (Chaps. 7, 8, and 9). We purposively do not make promises about classes being a "safe space" because avoiding all discomfort is both impossible and not even necessarily desirable. Our goal is to make the class "safe enough" in that MMP teachers make every effort to model a nonjudgmental stance and ensure that all opinions and experiences are respected by group members. While all agree to respect double confidentiality in the first class, the teacher cannot promise or enforce this agreement once students have left the classroom.

What Kind of Teacher/Teaching Style Is Most Helpful?

While some elements of MMP are essential (e.g., duration of each class and of the course, class size, uninterrupted class time, no laptops/cellphones), there is much within each class that is adaptable to the needs and skills of teachers and students across diverse areas. As has been noted earlier, *how* the learning exercises are taught is the most important element in making learning "stick." The "how" of teaching is related to the personal style of each teacher, and different approaches resonate with different students depending on their learning preferences. Small group teaching styles can vary from the teacher who prefers a contained pace and is more in control of which students speak and for how long, while other teachers are comfortable with a less-structured class atmosphere. Some teachers are comfortable asking questions of individual students in the large group setting, while others encourage participation but do not call on specific students. Some teachers find it helpful to bring in their own examples of what is being taught that relates to their own clinical encounters, while other teachers prefer to have the students themselves find their own clinical relevance. The exact balance between what is offered to students and what is being asked of them is an individual teaching style decision. There is no one way to teach MMP because there is no one type of student learner, and thus a heterogeneity of teaching styles is both inevitable and ultimately desirable.

Who Can Teach MMP?

An MMP teacher is a learner who is themselves a bit further along the path from not knowing to actualizing than the students they are teaching. Our MMP course is a mandatory requirement for McGill medical students created with the explicit intention of teaching essential clinical skills as outlined in the program learning objectives of the official curriculum. Because all students must complete MMP in order to graduate from McGill Medical School, we have found that those that teach MMP must have their own clinical expertise in order to bring "real-life" authentic clinical experience into the MMP classroom. Having experienced clinicians teach MMP gives the message that what is being taught in MMP is essential in the practice of clinical medicine and is not instead about "self-care" or "wellness", topics that students tend to associate with elective courses. We think that there is no more important message to the value of MMP in becoming a "good doctor" than having students see for themselves how practicing physicians relate each of the classes to their own clinical experiences.

How Much Meditation Experience Is Required?

Our MMP teachers have a range of previous meditative/contemplative practice, from extensive mindfulness-based stress reduction (MBSR) course and retreat experience over decades, to those who have only taken the 8-week MBSR course.

Some of our teachers have a regular personal meditation practice while others do not. As outlined in the teacher training section below, no matter the previous level of experience, all potential teachers go through a multistep vetting process that includes direct observation of their capacity to lead small groups, including guided awareness practices.

How to Develop an MMP Teacher

If we want to grow as teachers -- we must do something alien to academic culture: we must talk to each other about our inner lives -- risky stuff in a profession that fears the personal and seeks safety in the technical, the distant, the abstract. – Parker J. Palmer, from *The Courage to Teach: Exploring the Inner Landscape of a Teacher's Life*

For almost 2 hours, the MMP teacher is seated in a circle with 20 medical students, each with their own personal and cultural backgrounds and biases and preconceptions, with no slides, lectern, desk, or textbooks to hide behind or fall back upon. What the MMP teacher does have in hand is a one-page outline of the specific class activities and their own openness to bringing the material to life. The skilled teacher will use personal examples from their own life and clinical work sparingly, and with a clear intention of facilitating students' ability to connect to what is being taught with their own life and clinical experiences. Teaching MMP is, as one colleague put it, the "best and most challenging teaching I have ever done."

There are three additional prerequisites to becoming an MMP teacher, that include skills and experience:

1. Being a physician in the clinical practice of medicine
2. Teaching small groups
3. Guiding contemplative practices

We have found that the successful recruitment and training of MMP teachers follows the sequence of a four-step process that progresses from observation to increasing teaching responsibility and autonomy.

- *Step 1*: *Identifying the potential MMP teacher and a face-to-face meeting*. The first step in becoming an MMP teacher is explored in a face-to-face conversation between the potential teacher and the MMP course director(s). Issues to be discussed include ensuring that the MMP teacher has the required prerequisites and that they understand and agree with the vetting/training process and time commitments involved.
- *Step 2*: *Observation of one complete MMP course (set of seven classes)*. The potential teacher is invited to observe a full set of classes together with an experienced MMP teacher. This includes giving the potential teacher access to all of the teacher preparation materials, as outlined in the seven class chapters of this book, in advance of each class. At this stage the potential teacher is not co-teaching but is rather observing the set of seven classes. We have found it helpful to advise students of the passive role the observer will take during the course; otherwise students may incorrectly assume that the potential teacher is not being

given a voice rather than having agreed to the passive observer role. The post-class teacher debriefs (see next section "ongoing teacher support") are particularly important at this early stage in recruitment.

- *Step 3*: *Co-teaching a set of seven classes with an experienced teacher.* Co-teaching a set of seven MMP classes requires advance planning and deciding before each class which teacher will be responsible for teaching each class exercise. Before each class the two teachers meet to divide up the teaching responsibilities so that only one teacher is ever responsible for teaching a particular exercise. Beginning teachers may choose the specific exercises that they feel most comfortable with for the first few classes. For example, for some teachers leading a guided meditation is something they are comfortable with, and they may choose to do these exercises for the first classes. For others, guiding meditations may be more challenging, and they may choose to lead these only in later classes. As the course progresses, the new co-teacher should be encouraged and supported to teach at least 50% of each class and to specifically teach those exercises that they are less comfortable with.
- *Step 4*: *Teaching a set of seven classes independently.* Teaching alone (without a co-teacher) may not be the final step for all teachers. Some may find that co-teaching fits better for them, and if that is the case, then they may continue to co-teach over time.

Ongoing Teacher Support: Post-Class Debriefing

In the four-step process of recruiting a new teacher that takes 6–12 months, there is much opportunity for one-on-one coaching and mentoring. We have found it invaluable to ensure that after each class, there is 15–30 minutes of time set aside for teachers to meet together to debrief, and new teachers are expected to participate. Teaching the 1.5–2-hour class is demanding, and there are inevitably classes where the teacher will be energized and have a clear sense of having had a positive impact on students. At other times, there may be periods of doubt and regret about things said or not said within class. The post-class debrief is an opportunity to examine some of these issues and serves as both support and a source of ongoing learning for the teachers themselves. The post-class debrief is in some ways akin to a class itself, wherein mindful and sensitive exploration of issues that came up for each teacher can be raised and alternative interpretations of the meaning of what occurred in class explored. The debrief can be led by one teacher or may be a shared responsibility. What is important is that each teacher is given a non-judgmental space to reflect upon their teaching experience. We use a debriefing format of going in order from one exercise to the next in sequence for each class and allowing space for each teacher to speak in turn about what went well and what did not go well for each exercise. Teachers have also benefitted from sharing different styles and ways of responding to commonly encountered difficult issues that arise over the course (e.g., ways to respond to what appears to be a bored or angry student).

Assessment and Evaluation of Students

The specific methods used to assess students during MMP will depend upon the individual medical school's existing grading requirements. Students in MMP should be assessed with the same methods used for other mandatory courses they are required to pass. Our McGill MMP course occurs within the pre-clerkship 6-month period of three 8-week blocks. There are three separate student assessments, and each is required to be passed in order to pass the course.

1. *Multiple-choice questions*: At the end of each 8-week pre-clerkship block (that includes other courses such as a medical ethics course as well as pre-clerkship medical and surgical hospital rotations), there is a multiple-choice exam that covers all the rotations and courses in that particular block. MMP is assessed in the same way as these other courses within each block – there are multiple-choice questions (MCQs) we have created to assess students' understanding of the more cognitive concepts embedded in MMP. Such concepts include the definition of terms (e.g., mindfulness) and concepts (e.g., the different Satir stances). The content of the MCQs is derived from MMP class objectives, and there are ten MMP MCQs per exam.
2. *Class participation and engagement*: Students are assessed by each MMP teacher using an assessment form similar to that used for the pre-clinical medicine and surgical rotations. The modified assessment form has sections for teachers to evaluate each student's participation, engagement, and group contribution on a pass/fail basis.
3. *Essays*: During the last (seventh) class of each block, students are assigned a reflective written essay that is due to be handed in 1 week later (see Chap. 12). The essay has two parts and asks them to describe their experience of participating in the course in a maximum of 500 words and also to outline which and why specific class themes and exercises may be particularly helpful in their future clinical practice in no more than 750 words (see Chap. 9, Class 7). A grade of 60% is required to pass the essay.

We advise students that we (each MMP teacher) will personally read each essay and offer written feedback, and that we take what they write seriously. We tell students that we are looking for honest reflections on what they have learned during the course. We have found the written assignment to be useful first as a way to consolidate learning, as students need to review each class exercise in order to write the essay (and they have the class notes in Appendix F to help them do this). Second, we have found the essay helpful in revealing the wide range of responses to the question of what they found will be potentially useful in their future practice. Reading the essays of hundreds of students over the past 4 years, we have found that:

- There are frequently directly opposing examples of what students like and do not like and find helpful and unhelpful in the course. For example, as many students comment on not appreciating being asked to share their experiences in the dyad exercises as those who find these interactions to be the most helpful. There are also about equal numbers of students who find the contemplative exercises helpful as those who struggle with them.

- Student essays range from those that are highly thoughtful and reflective to those that are more superficial, and this allows for grading that typically ranges from 60% to 100%.
- There are significant numbers of students who are relatively quiet in class, but whose essays demonstrate a deep understanding of the learning objectives.
- There is often a very small number of students who struggle with personal issues that make specific exercises and classes difficult for them.
- The most common theme is that of the student who was skeptical at first but saw for themselves the value of the course as classes progressed.

Criteria to Pass the Course

In order to pass the course, students are required to:

1. Attend at least six out of the seven classes. If they miss/do not attend more than one class (i.e., if they attend less than six of the seven classes), they are assigned a "makeup" assignment that includes readings and a reflective writing paper based on the reading that is to be handed in 1 week before they then need to meet with their MMP teacher and present their paper. Because of the pedological imperative to make available to students the capacity to "make up" more than one missed class, we have reluctantly created this makeup assignment, but we do not think it adequately addresses the issue that an MMP class is essentially not replaceable. The learning that occurs within each MMP class is a co-created process that emerges from the specific small group dynamic that has been built up class by class and cannot be recreated by separate individual assignments. If students miss more than one class, we require them to retake the full set of seven classes the next time they are offered. We advise students of the limitations inherent in makeup assignments, and we articulate how they are a less than satisfactory solution. We also remind students that in MMP class, "to be late is to miss a class" and that they need to plan carefully for missed buses, inclement weather, malfunctioning alarm clocks, and any other reasons why they may struggle to get to class before the door closes. We have found that making these issues clear in the first class has resulted in very few times when a makeup class has been necessary.

2. Receive a "pass" on the class participation and engagement evaluation form that the teacher completes for each student. Should a student show a lack of participation or be presenting difficulties within the in-class group dynamic, we address these issues first with the student and then with the Dean of Undergraduate Medical Education when appropriate, well before the end of the course. With this system of identifying students with difficulties early on in the course and with early intervention, we have not failed a student at this point in time based on this part of the evaluation.

3. Pass the essay with a grade of at least 60%.
4. Receive a grade of at least 60% on the end-of-the-block MCQ exam. We advise students that MMP MCQs are based on the pre-prepared class notes and that if they have attended classes and read the notes, then they should not have difficulty answering the MCQs correctly. It is not uncommon to have many students answer 100% of the MMP MCQ exam questions correctly, and that is the outcome we hope for. The conceptual knowledge required to pass the MCQs is the least important aspect of what we hope students will learn from the course. It is very rare to have a student receive a grade of less than 60% on the MCQ exam. Should they receive a grade of less than 60%, they have the opportunity to retake the exam with a different set of questions.

References

1. Bone RC. The taste of lemonade on a summer afternoon. JAMA. 1995;273(7):518. https://doi. org/10.1001/jama.1995.03520310010003.
2. Krasner MS, Epstein RM, Beckman H, Suchman AL, Chapman B, Mooney CJ, et al. Association of an educational program in mindful communication with burnout, empathy, and attitudes among primary care physicians. JAMA. 2009;302(12):1284–93. https://doi. org/10.1001/jama.2009.1384.

Chapter 12
End-of-Course Essays: Students' Responses to the Course

Tom A. Hutchinson

At the conclusion of the Mindful Medical Practice (MMP) course, students are asked to write an essay that includes 500 words on their experience participating in the MMP course. We asked 20 students comprising the complete group taught by Drs. Tom Hutchinson and John Hoffer in the most recent iteration of the course (January 11 to February 22, 2019) for permission to use their essay in our book. This request was made after the essays had been submitted, marked, and commented on. Students were not aware this request would be made at the time they wrote their essay. Eighteen students complied. Below are their unedited comments.

Student 1

Two months ago, my classmates and I showed up at New Residence Hall, excited to hear about the next step of our medical school journey: TCP. It was our first-day orientation, and in the span of about 7 hours, we received information from various course directors and administrators about what to expect as assignments and assessments. Towards the end of the internal medicine block presentation, a professor walked towards our class and, without a microphone, stood between us and introduced us to the Mindful Medical Practice course. He stood between all of the students and told us that every year, students get mistaken and think that MMP will be about our own personal wellness. He made sure to let us know, and convincingly so, that the course was about much more than that. We were to be challenged and pushed to think beyond our usual thoughts and concerns. Considering the impactful introduction to the course and my subsequent memorable experience, I was surprised by the fact that this was the first time I ever heard about MMP and that it wasn't brought up more often by upper year students when speaking to my class about their TCP experience.

S. Liben, T. A. Hutchinson, *MD Aware*,
https://doi.org/10.1007/978-3-030-22430-1_12

Honestly, I had yet to experience a course like MMP before these past few months. When I stepped into McIntyre's room 201 and saw chairs placed in a circle, I was a bit confused about what was to come. Dr. X quickly explained the course and gave the group an overview of what we should expect. Looking around, I was a bit relieved to see that none of my close friends were in my group. I knew most of the students around me, but most were acquaintances. I believe this allowed my MMP experience to be more honest and impactful on my own take on mindfulness. Surprisingly, it made discussing my feelings and beliefs easier because I didn't feel that anyone would compare what I was saying with how I usually act. In other words, I felt I could express myself truly, without putting up a brave face or being fearful that someone may relate my words with what may be going on in my personal life. I also find it important to note how much I appreciated the way Dr. X reiterated to the group that all discussions were to be kept confidential and that our group was a safe space for honest discussion. So many of my classmates opened up, more so towards the end of the course, whether it be because we developed a certain level of trust between us or because the exercises we went through helped us word our thoughts and concerns more easily.

I am usually one to laugh when confronted with emotional discussions. We were asked to really try to move past laughter and such reactions early on in the exercises as a way to take the lessons of MMP more seriously. Being told to do so by the professor made the course more real. In fact, the easiest way to approach emotions and heavy topics is to take them "à la légère" and laugh through them. To take a moment to get past the sometimes difficult task of initiating honest conversation made me actually reflect on the different topics presented and get through the tasks on my own. Being repeatedly paired up with Dr. Y in most of the exercises made me want to resort to laughing as a response to serious questions and to get away from nervous feelings related to sharing personal details with a teacher; however he was so willing to share his own experiences that I felt a lot more comfortable as classes went on.

I hope the MMP experience will continue to be offered to all medical students in TCP, an opportune time of transition to discuss a mindful approach to clinical practice.

Student 2

My experience in participating in the Mindful Medical Practice course was overall very enriching, to say the least.

I found it very interesting that it put forward, among others, a different approach to teaching than our other courses in the curriculum. Although this might seem a bit innocuous, being myself someone who is very organized in terms of my school material and that has a tendency to take overly detailed notes during classes – which a lot of the time prevents me from capturing the overall messages and ideas that a lecture wishes to deliver – I particularly appreciated that no electronic devices and computers were allowed and that a lot of the planned activities were very interactive, as it genuinely allowed me to capture the true essence of this course. I found that I was better able to learn and to understand the different concepts and theories, and surprisingly I was much more focused on the class and retained more information than usual.

I also appreciated how every exercise done or topic discussed was always brought back, by the teachers, to how they could be applied to our future clinical practice and to our current interactions with patients. The fact that this correlation between meditative/mindful practices and the medical field was always very clear made it very interesting as I learned more about essential communication and awareness skills that are beneficial to both clinicians and students, despite them not necessarily being explicitly taught in formal lectures.

I was always looking forwards to going to the small group sessions every Friday morning. It was such a nice way to end the week. I must admit however that some classes (like "Class 6 – Being with Suffering") did trigger a high level of anxiety within myself and that sometimes, activities made me dig so deep into my thoughts and left myself questioning a lot about my goals and what values are truly important to me, to the point where it made me feel uncomfortable. I now realize, however, that it is part of the process of becoming a better person and developing a healthier mindset, and I absolutely don't consider these instances as being "downsides" of this course!

Furthermore, I very much appreciated how the supervisors did an excellent job in making the class a safe environment for students to open up about their experiences and to deliver their opinions in a judgement-free space. It put me very much at ease to participate more, which in turn contributed in making my experience more enjoyable. I had the opportunity to be exposed to perspectives about certain subjects that I have never thought of before, and it allowed my knowledge and open-mindedness to be broadened to a great extent. I was very thankful for this aspect of the class.

All in all, personally, the Mindful Medical Practice class truly reached its goal as I now know more of ways to better care for patients as well as for myself. This course allowed me to efficiently practice specific listening skills, to change my perception of certain social and communication behaviors that I have, and also to simply be more aware of my very own person, of my tendencies to act in certain situations, and of how to deal with my attitude in cases where it might interfere negatively with my professional and personal relationships.

Student 3

The Mindfulness and Medical Practice course greatly surpassed my expectations. In total honesty, I initially did not think that this class would change so importantly the way I envision my future medical practice and even the way I deal with problems and adversity in my daily life. Throughout my entire education, not only in medical school, I had been exposed to similar classes and formations, but they had never left me with much to carry on with. I think one of the factors that made this class different from what I experienced before is how brilliantly the tutors were able to lead our journey into mindfulness and congruent thinking by being completely understanding, open-minded, and nonjudgmental. I am grateful to have had tutors that had all of the right qualities to run such a sensitive and sometimes very emotionally charged class and to have shared with us their wisdom and, at times, very morally challenging experiences. Another important factor that played a role in my positive experience taking this class is also the group I was assigned to. Indeed, a lot of students in the group were willing to openly share moments of their life that were most of the time personal or difficult to share. This was very helpful for other students to learn from their situation or even just to relate to their problem and to be able to feel like we're not the only one living a similar situation. Of course, the fact that the rest of the group was also always receptive, as well as open-minded and nonjudgmental, was an important player in the success of our sharing circle. The safe environment that was provided through this course is a unique setting where everyone was comfortable with sharing, and that setting is not easy to obtain, but all of the factors named before made it possible. It permitted the group to learn from each other and understand how each person's past experiences and background shaped us in the people we are today. Lastly, what really most importantly made a difference from other similar experiences I was exposed to before is the fact that I was mature enough and aware enough of myself, my own experiences, my own longings, and my own fears to be able to introspect and move forward. When I had a similar class in high school, no one ever took it seriously because we were all, without even knowing it, too immature and too far from our emotions to make the most out of it. I personally didn't share that many of my experiences or opinions to the group, mainly because English is not my first language and I've always been self-conscious about speaking in a group or for a presentation in English. I hope this wasn't seen badly by making other people feel like I didn't care or wasn't interested in the course, because I was. I also am a more private person, and after every class, I enjoyed talking about every exercise or concept we've been through in class with my closer group of friends rather than to the group that consisted of many people I've never talked to before. Overall, my experience was completely positive, and hopefully, I think most of the students that will go through this course will feel the same as me.

Student 4

The Mindful Medical Practice course was a moment of reprieve in otherwise hectic weeks. In a medical curriculum seemingly lacking in humanities and the "soft skills" of medicine, taking the time each week to take a step back and reflect on patient interactions, student experiences, reactions, and expectations of medicine was welcome. The course setting (sitting in a circle, without taking notes or being distracted by devices) made it even more impactful, as it forced students to be in the present moment. With course work, studying and the use of UpToDate requiring us to use our computers all the time, it is quite rare that medical students get the opportunity to totally disconnect.

After completing the Fundamentals of Medicine and Dentistry portion of our training, I had a discussion with a first-year resident and friend about how closely our grades in the first 2 years of medical school related to our performance in clerkship. His conclusion was that medicine was as much about treating illnesses as it was about supporting our patients and having an excellent bedside manner; the human side of medicine was what distinguished good clerks from great ones. But in an environment where healthcare professionals are overworked and burnt-out, taking the time to be mindful of the patients' experience is underemphasized. This course was helpful in guiding us from the beginning on strategies to be more mindful in practice and recognizing the importance of approaching each case as a doctor-patient partnership and "healthy" as meaning more than just "disease-free."

To me, the most valuable aspect of the course was creating a space where all students could share their thoughts and concerns without judgment. As the weeks went on and my peers became more familiar with each other and the course structure, I was pleasantly surprised to see that more and more students were sharing their personal stories and emotions. Up until now, there hadn't been many venues – and even fewer structured ones – for students to discuss their struggles. There were several times during MMP that a student commented on the fact that it seemed that everyone felt the same way (effectively mitigating "imposter syndrome") and although this isn't a wellness class, I think the course's contribution to student wellness should nonetheless be noted.

Furthermore, the timing of the class within the curriculum was perfect. As we started seeing patients and witnessing the day-to-day responsibilities of the clerks and residents, it left many students with thoughts and feelings that were then addressed or discussed on Friday mornings. Discussing meditation techniques or our approach to suffering during this part of our training, for example, had added value because it related back to many of the first-time experiences we were having at the hospital. Other topics, such as clinical congruence, helped us think critically of the bedside manner of our staff.

In the world of medicine, where the bar is set close to perfection, the pressure is high, and students are constantly competing, taking a step back, pausing, and re-centering ourselves around what really matters was incredibly valuable.

Student 5

I was very skeptical going into the first mindfulness session we had at the beginning of TCP. I thought "I don't need this," "I would rather have these few extra hours to sleep or study or read," "This is a waste of time," etc. The first session started with a meditation exercise. I had tried to meditate in the past, through online applications or videos, which was always "unsuccessful." I was always doing something "wrong." I thought that perhaps doing it in a group, in the setting of a course with a mediator in the room would help me meditate "right." It took a few mindfulness sessions for me to realize that there is no right or wrong way to meditate. The point was not to clear my thoughts and focus on a specific body part or breathing cycle, but to be aware of my thoughts and be okay with having them, instead of fighting to push them away. The point of meditation was to be mindful. Although this realization helped me understand that I was not meditating wrong in the past, which made me feel less guilty, it did not make me want to do it more often. Personally, meditation does not help reduce my stress or anxiety. I understand that it can be very helpful for others, who truly enjoyed this part of the course. I continuously tried to meditate and to enjoy it throughout the sessions, but it did not help, which I don't blame myself for anymore. It is good to know what coping strategies help or don't help because they can be very different for each individual – as long as they are healthy coping strategies. Personally, talking about our experiences and discussing stressful events with a group help me, which was a great element in this course.

Being in a room full of friends, acquaintances, and even strangers, going through similar experiences, listening to your thoughts and relating to your stories made me feel very grateful. It made me realize that I am not alone on this journey and that everyone has their own bumps on that road. Seeing that made me feel less lonely and made me realize that I can talk about these bumps more openly than I thought I could, without being judged. Even the people who I thought had everything together, and were never stressed and never worried, turned out to be more similar to me than I thought. It was a great safe space to talk about our fears, worries, and stressful events but also discuss positive experiences and share different ways to cope with different emotions. I enjoyed the discussion parts of the course, as this is my usual method of decreasing stress and anxiety. I like to talk about things and hear other people's experiences to know that I am not going through them alone and that you can get through it and it gets better.

At the last session of MMP, I was glad this course was integrated in TCP and happy I got to meet new people from class, realize that we're all going through this together, and see another side of medical students that we don't always like to show.

Student 6

My experience with the Mindful Medical Practice course has been a good reinforcement of my personal practices for the last 4 years. For the most part, the concepts in the course were not new to me. I have personally studied self-development continuously through reading books by prominent authors such as Robin Sharma, Tony Robbins, and Brandon Bouchard. I continuously consume podcasts which discuss themes that we encountered during Mindful Medical Practice. It was very interesting to watch the other members of my class discuss these subjects and listening to the various opinion. I feel that our group was probably the most engaged, likely due to the fact that the majority of the group consisted of female students. I do not make that conjecture from the place of sexist prejudice. It is true that women are more in tune with emotion and have greater emotional maturity and capacity. It becomes very difficult if one has to engage in discussing the subjects in this course without a baseline level of emotional maturity. I must point out though that the few male classmates were fairly engaged and I was very impressed by their level of attention. I personally had several roadblocks when it came to sharing personal knowledge and experience. First and foremost, I am new to the class, and thus my comfort level with those around me was not optimal no matter how "safe" the space was. I also did not want to seem as an individual who has been learning in the background as I soon realized that this was not the norm of the cohort. This did not surprise me; I'm well aware that most of the world are uninterested in the prospect that self-help can make a difference and improve their lives. My intention was not to stand out, and thus I refrained from sharing on several occasions even though I had something to say to the group. During activities where one was to share one's own experience to another classmate, I often opted to share a more benign story although I had a more personal matter that was more fitting. I never felt like I was being judged, but still I was not comfortable sharing to someone that I did not know on a personal level. The other activities and meditations were very helpful. I would always start the activity with a sense of wonder thinking what exactly is being taught. By the end, it always became apparent that the activity was a proxy for the overall theme of the day.

Student 7

When we first got our TCP schedules, I saw I had MMP every Friday morning. I was actually annoyed we had to attend and thought that this would be a waste of my time. I wanted to be in the hospital as much as possible and not in class. Previous TCP students told me that if I was late to class, I was not allowed in. I was told that we would spend hours talking about our emotions and concentrating on our body parts. Needless to say, I already had a preconceived opinion of this class, and I was not excited to attend it. Little did I know how much this class was going to be helpful. Here we are, 8 weeks after our very first class, and I am so grateful we had this opportunity. I ended up learning a lot of valuable lessons that I am certain will help me to become a better physician. I learned how to be more aware of my own feelings and I realized that I hate facing them. I learned that I have the tendency to be super-reasonable to avoid facing my emotions and feelings. I learned that sometimes it is important to take a step back and breathe in order to come up with the best solution and see the big picture. Most importantly I learned how to become more aware of my surroundings and have become a better listener, which will help me become the best physician I can be.

As a medical student, I am constantly busy: whether it is studying, being part of charity events, or being involved in the student council. I used to feel guilty when I was taking time for myself. The first meditation class we had made me uncomfortable. Ironically, sitting in silence to meditate made me anxious. I was unable to focus, I was moving my legs, and my mind was spinning at a thousand miles an hour. However, as the weeks went by, I felt less anxious about sitting in silence; I was less distracted and was even able to realize when my mind was elsewhere. I was also anxious about some group activities. I was surrounded by so many people I had never spoken to. I was struggling opening up to my classmates and did not want to share personal stories. But as the weeks went by, I felt more comfortable sharing stories. I learned how to listen to my classmates, and I realized how wonderful they were. I think the most important lesson I learned was that "I am not alone." I felt we were all here to support and help each other and it was a wonderful feeling.

Finally, I really enjoyed the Mindful Medical Practice class. I am very grateful to have had this class at the very start of my clinical journey. It taught me things that we were never taught in class or small groups. I loved interacting with my peers and I enjoyed the way the class was taught. It was a big change from the usual didactic lectures we are used to get in medicine. I opened up more than I ever thought I would and I learned so much about myself. I ended up learning valuable lessons that will help me become the most congruent physician I could be.

Student 8

The Doubt

Starting out 8 weeks ago, I did not really know what to expect from the Mindful Medical Practice course. Friends in more senior years of medical school mentioned that the course was relaxing, was a nice way to end the week, and involved some meditation. I was curious to find out what exactly was meant by meditation, as this practice can take many forms. I was also interested to find out what was meant by mindfulness, as in my experience, this term is sometimes misused to simply refer to anything new age or hippie, without a real appreciation for, and implementation of, mindfulness in everyday life.

My previous experiences with meditation and the cultivation of mindfulness also brought old baggage, old disappointment in myself, and old biases. To give a little context, I have had a few periods in my life when I was travelling and stumbled into communities that focused on meditative practices for various reasons. Some hippie communities off the grid in Hawaii preached meditation and mindfulness as a way to build a better world, but I often felt that they were just hiding from regret and past mistakes. Tree planters in the interior of British Columbia seemed to use it to get through the harsh cold and hard, long work.

A particularly intense period of personal practice was when I lived for a month and a half in Wat Pho, a Buddhist monastery in Thailand's second city, as an active part of the songha or community. Here I finally felt that the monks around me were on to something real, and although I could not understand all of their teachings, the pursuit of personal betterment, purposeful action, and compassionate consideration for others was evident and palpable. But once I returned home to continue my university education, I felt that I quickly lost any ground that I had gained towards incorporating mindfulness into my everyday life.

When I heard that we were going to be meditating with a doctor on the second floor of McIntyre Medical Building along with all of the other type A medical student personalities, I just really didn't know what to expect. How was this going to help me as a doctor? What kind of meditation we were going to do? Would the instructor be a new age hippie, a workaholic imposter, or a truly genuine practitioner that could reignite an appreciation for taking a little extra time to breathe, contemplate, and consider? Unfortunately, I allowed my ego to creep into the picture and offered doubts regarding the usefulness of these Friday morning sessions.

The Reality

This course was well structured, well delivered, and well received by myself and my classmates. The 5–10-minute guided meditation periods reminded me of the utility of taking a minute to stop, reflect, breathe, and then move on to the next tasks at hand. The analogies presented throughout the course were poignant and constructive, and the constant links to medical practice made evident the value of this type of course, at this stage in our training.

It was not easy for me to reflect on things going on in my life, how I am handling stress or conflicts, my inner fears, or my outer expectations. This was compounded through the duration of the course by the fact that my life partner and main support system was far away in the Northwest Territories for work. But the openness of the class as well as the respect and humility of the instructor really facilitated reflective discussion in a safe and productive manner. I enjoyed the discussions around how to be a more thoughtful, considerate, and congruent clinician and hope to take these lessons in my future practice.

The meditation style was difficult for me. Trying to concentrate on just one thing at a time, be it a big toe or a breath, was nearly impossible for me, and I found myself constantly comparing it to other styles that I have practiced in the past. For instance, in the Theravada Buddhist Community that I was welcomed into in Thailand, they use a method of labelling to allow one to focus on everything that comes into the mind and then simply acknowledge its presence and let it pass as a new thought or feeling emerges. However, I appreciate that the technique of focusing on one aspect of our physical reality while attempting to let our thoughts come and go freely may be helpful later in our careers when we need to be conscious of the physical signs within our patients and ourselves.

Another difficulty for me was dealing with the negativity that was often overflowing throughout the sessions. It was clear that many of my classmates were dealing with immense fear and self-doubt about the next steps in our education, but the meetings often felt more like a therapy session than constructive discussions on how to cultivate mindfulness. But I too vented at times and appreciate that everyone deserves to be heard and give their opinions. I noticed, however, that response to the instructor's questions was often off topic and I sometimes would have appreciated a bit more pull back to the discussion point at hand.

Overall, I had a wonderful time during the Mindful Medical Practice course. I enjoyed and appreciated the insight offered by the tutor and was impressed with how well the activities were then related back to clinical problems and issues that often arise between physicians and patients, between physicians and other allied health professionals, and between physicians themselves and within themselves. This course offered real and tangible suggestions and solutions to how we can improve our future medical practice for the benefit of our patients and ourselves.

Student 9

It was a pleasure to participate in the MMP courses these last few weeks. Each class built on the others to give us a better understanding of how to be more mindful and congruent not only in our future clinical practice but also in our daily lives so that we may be more empathetic and well-rounded people. This class gave me a better perspective on how to have more meaningful connections with my family and friends, and, although it will be difficult to apply in the context of relationships with people I already know well, having these tools at my disposable can only benefit me.

I especially enjoyed the four stances as shown by the self, the other, and the context. The four stances allowed me to realize how I tend to take on the various stances in my daily life, and how when I have unsuccessful interactions with others, it is usually because the other person or myself are taking on a stance other than the congruent one. It also taught me to not judge or think negatively of myself or others when we take on one of these stances and simply try to bring the situation back to the present in a calm and serene way. I believe that this would especially be helpful in conflict resolution so that we may have more successful interactions with a greater number of people. It can also allow us to live better with ourselves and the situations we find ourselves in, even if these situations might be unpleasant. We now have a better way to deal with these situations and to understand those who disagree with us in a more respectful way.

I also really liked the iceberg exercise, which I think is a good summary for both the sessions on suffering and on mindful congruent practice in clerkship and beyond. I think that the exercise really demonstrates how everyone has the same longings and yearnings: we all want to have a fulfilled life and to be appreciated by those around us. It is our expectations, perceptions, and feelings that are different, and the stances that we take influence our surface personality and what others see in us. At the end of the day, when faced with our own mortality, everyone wants to make sure that their affairs are in order, that those they leave behind will be somewhat ok after they pass on, and that they have lived a life that is satisfying to them. Everyone we agree or disagree with has all felt the same fears and joys as us in the context of the deeper levels of the iceberg. Even if we might dislike what we see in some people on the surface level, this exercise allowed us to realize that this level is only a very small part of who they are and that everything they do is simply because they have the same longings and yearnings as ourselves.

I believe that this class has helped me gain a better understanding of not only myself, but of various situations I might find myself in. I really enjoyed how open people were willing to be with each other and how trustworthy people are about the confidentiality of the experiences we shared. I am grateful that I had the opportunity to participate in such a meaningful class.

Student 10

One of my first experiences in the Mindful Medical Practice course became the background for many of the thoughts and reflections that the course elicited over the 7 weeks that it ran. Before beginning the session with a guided meditation, our instructor mentioned that if, during the meditation, our attention wandered and got lost in a story, it would be appropriate to acknowledge that we had left the specific task of the meditation and to gently come back to the present moment. During the meditation, at a point where we were asked to focus our attention on our knee, a story came along and swept me away. Focusing on my knee reminded me that it was feeling mildly uncomfortable, which led me to think of my mom's side of the family who always said they had "bad knees" and think about my grandpa and my cousin who had both had knee replacements. Maybe I would need a knee replacement someday, or maybe bad knees are just a family legend and my knees are fine? At this point I gently acknowledged I was lost in a story and returned to focusing on my knee in the present moment. I would think back on this experience and how lucky I was to have a story like this! Focusing on something as simple as my knee took me straight away to thoughts of my mother, grandfather, and cousin – within my knee was a story, and that story connected me to people I love. How many more stories might be hiding in my knee? What stories might I find in my shoulder, my ears, or my ring finger? I was reminded of a quote from Thomas King's CBC Massey Lectures: "The truth about stories is that that's all we are" (2003). With this in mind, as I develop my skills as a physician, in all my interactions with patients, I think my main goal is to be attentive to my patients' stories, as well as to the stories I bring with me into any individual patient encounter. Together, both the patient and I will co-create a new story, a story we will share. Throughout the Mindful Medical Practice course, I developed new stories, stories that are personal but also ones that are collective, shared with my classmates and instructors. I would like to share now a few more of these stories about my experience in the class, how it challenged me and helped me to grow, and how its themes and exercises will continue to guide my development as a physician.

Student 11

My experiences in the MMP course have been surprisingly positive and productive. I am not sure what my expectations were coming into the curriculum, but they were most definitely surpassed. I appreciated the career insight provided to us by our group leaders. They always embodied patience while leading our open-ended discussions. This allowed the entire experience to flow genuinely. Each session did not feel forced or artificially structured. We were allowed the space to voice whatever it was that came to mind, and we were also gifted the opportunity to stay silent when it suited us better. I appreciated that each session revolved around a theme, one that we weren't all necessarily aware of. I believe that this really did help structure the dialogue and dyad conversations in a way that never felt redundant.

Our MMP course experience was successful for a number of reasons, but I do give a lot of credit and gratitude to the openness and honesty of our group. Even though we are all in our second year together, I cannot say that I know most of my colleagues very well. While we chitchat about school and rotations, nothing usually stems much deeper in conversation unless I have a relationship with a friend outside the classroom. For this reason, I was surprised, if not inspired, by how much my peers were willing to share with us. It also further allowed me to speak my mind and feel comfortable doing so. I have always been very good and comfortable listening to other people. Ironically, as open and honest as I feel like I am with both myself and other people, I have always struggled with sharing more of me than is asked. It is not that I am closed off; I suppose I am just guarded to share more of myself than I need to. This might be because I have taught myself not to dwell on the things that get me down. I do not usually complain, nor do I engage in the usual social engagement of being bonded through our woes. For this reason, I sometimes feel as though I am on the outside of the group social network of my peers.

It was extremely touching for me to hear about the feelings and experiences of people who I was only vaguely familiar with. It allowed me to understand that we are all connected in more ways that I previously thought. It is always empowering to realize that you are part of something bigger than yourself, especially during those times where you think that you are dealing with something all alone. I also noticed something interesting: I was less likely to speak up when I disagreed with someone. Perhaps this was in the spirit of kinship and me not wanting to dampen the overall group vibe. I of course never wanted anyone to feel as though what they were saying did not have merit, so if I did not choose my words correctly, it could potentially risk the whole dynamic of the group. This way, if I were to disagree with what was being said, I would instead voice my opinion and perspective in a way that simply came across as adding another idea to the table. I think it was important that we not see the MMP sessions as a debate and more so as a round table of open-ended discussion that was thought provoking, inclusive, and a safe space to share anything. I think it requires maturity to be able to speak your mind but also to know when staying silent is more appropriate. Sometimes it is not about you and it is indeed someone else's moment. We, as professionals going into the business of interacting with people at their most vulnerable, need to know how to master the skill of social awareness and emotional intelligence. In the end, it was really beautiful to see us come together every Friday and unload or reflect on the challenges and fears that we all face. It has had both a calming and empowering effect on me as a student, and I really appreciated the experience at this stage in my medical career.

Student 12

I am grateful to have had the opportunity to participate in the MMP course. I think that its structure and topics have provided for very interesting and enlightening Friday mornings for our class. I don't believe that many of us knew what this course would be like, and as a result, I had very few expectations for it in the first place. However, this course turned out to be very thought provoking and stimulating in a way that few other courses have been for me before. Through authentic, vulnerable, and meaningful group discussions, we have touched on many challenging topics, from suffering to resilience, that have all taught us to pause and reflect in our day-to-day lives. I believe that this course sparked a new level of thoughtfulness in us all, and I found myself walking out of the class every week feeling grateful to have taken part.

In this course, we have explored our fears, concerns, and insecurities in an open and honest way. I am grateful that our group especially was so willing to participate and divulge personal information and experiences. This made me feel closer to them as colleagues, as I was able to see how many of us share such similar challenges but also see how different everyone's individual experiences are. Given the huge undertaking that we have all taken on as medical trainees, I believe that having a sense of community and belonging is very important. We will inevitably all face significant challenges in this journey, and without a support system that is able to relate and empathize with us, this experience would be that much more challenging. I am hopeful that this openness will continue to inspire us to reach out to each other for support in the future.

In a way, this course has also helped me to develop more respect for my colleagues as future clinicians as well, seeing how honest my classmates were in the sometimes very challenging discussions we had. If we consider the role of the doctor as a healer of the physical, psychological, and spiritual aspects of a patient's life, I think that it becomes especially important for physicians to be in tune with their own mental well-being as well as the impact of their words and actions on others. It is important for us to develop the ability to pause and reflect on our feelings towards things before we act on them, and this requires a certain amount of self-awareness. Seeing my colleagues respond to the various activities and discussions in such an open and vulnerable way showed me how seriously everyone takes their job as a future healer and how honestly everyone hoped to benefit from the lessons being taught. This willingness to learn from self-evaluation I believe is a very important skill, and I often felt humbled to see how seriously my colleagues took this undertaking.

Overall, this experience helped me to reflect on and evaluate my feelings and actions towards others as well as myself. It also showed me how thoughtfully and genuinely my colleagues did the same thing, which I was grateful to have participated in. I think that the class was placed at an opportune time, just as we are all beginning to enter the clinics and experience patients for the first time. I am grateful for the genuine discussions, to my colleagues for participating, and to Dr. X for creating such an open and comfortable space for it to all take place in.

Student 13

My experience participating in the MMP course was very interesting because I felt like I was able to truly reflect on my experiences in medicine and it revealed a lot. Coming to the class every Friday morning was actually a very rewarding thing as I felt that, as a class, we were able to connect and get to know each other in a safe environment. Initially, I was not sure what to expect from this class as it was a bit vague and I actually thought it was going to be in a lecture format. At the beginning, I thought it would be a bit of a challenge to constantly be engaged in the conversation as opposed to a lecture format where I could just focus on the subject and learn the "facts." Ironically, this kind of format of a class, where we could discuss in a group setting and sit in a circle without any distractions such as using a computer, was one of the most rewarding and engaging courses I have ever been in. I felt like the weekly meetings were very therapeutic in addition to highly interesting and of course very useful. The various aspects of this class were combined in interesting ways through the use of activities that truly allowed us as students to experience these realizations rather than just being told what they were. Some of the realizations I had in these past 8 weeks include thinking more about my patients' point of view and trying to be more in the moment. I have a tendency to rush and try to always think ahead, and, in a way, I realized through this class that I am always worrying about what will happen next, and in doing this, I am missing out on things occurring in the present and also missing out on connecting with the others around me. Having these realizations has helped me experience the hospital setting in TCP more fully and have helped me take a pause when I feel overwhelmed. I think this course has enabled me to become more attuned to what I may experience in the future as a physician as well as the challenges my colleagues may face, as there are increasing amounts of burnout and issues with mental health among this field of work. I think that through my experience in taking this course, I have also become more attuned to my classmates and feel like I am able to better relate to them. The dynamic of our group was so welcoming and nurturing, and I believe that it provided a moment of relief among our busy lives. I know that many of my classmates, including myself, felt this sense of relief because in general we are all very competitive and are always comparing ourselves to each other. It helped to know that, despite being in an environment of extreme competitiveness, we are all experiencing similar challenges and obstacles and that we are not isolated in these feelings.

Student 14

I honestly don't remember what I was expecting when I entered the classroom the first day of class. If anything, I was stressed out because I was late, because I had slept past my alarms, because I had probably missed the bus and the subway, and because I had just stressfully power walked up the hill in order to get to class. (As I'm typing this, I'm feeling a surge of stress.) In hindsight, I think it was very fitting that I was in such a state when I was first introduced to the course on mindfulness. Getting to class – something that could have been (should have been?) a simple commute, an everyday thing – was overwhelmingly stressful, because of the way that I assigned meaning to being late. I dwelled on how fatigued I was, how I was going to miss the beginning of the class and then somehow not pay attention to the rest of it, how my schedule always felt out of my control, how I was never going to survive clerkship if I couldn't even make it to a 9 AM class, and how I was maybe just intrinsically lazy and not meant for a career in medicine. I'll be honest: this is how many of my mornings would start. Sometimes it would lead to a day of laziness because I would give up before 10 AM; sometimes it would lead to a day of productivity if I somehow managed to white-knuckle through things out of stress.

The MMP course was different because even though most of the course's classes started with mornings that fit the description above, I usually left feeling better. I found it easy to pay attention to and be engaged in, even on the days where my fatigue felt insurmountable, and I couldn't imagine dragging myself out of bed. I wouldn't say that the course was life-changing or that it taught me something that I hadn't heard of before, but it definitely primed my day and weekend in a way that I found to be subtle but powerful nonetheless. At first I thought it was the content, because I was being reminded of the ways that mindfulness and emotional awareness could benefit my life, but it wasn't just that; I realized with each class that it was the sense of community that I found to be the most beneficial… and therapeutic, even? The way that the course was set up truly encouraged the group to be thoughtful and genuine with their answers. As such, listening to my colleagues openly talk truly did strike me. I didn't personally know each and every one of my classmates going in, and yet, when they spoke about their thought patterns, their concerns, and fears, I found that most things that were being said resonated deeply within me. It was like my thoughts were being put into other people's words, and I found a true sense of comfort in that. The best way to put it is that each class reminded me that I wasn't the only one having a difficult morning when I was having a difficult morning.

Of course, I think the inevitable reality is that a lot of mornings will continue to be difficult – fatigue and stress will always be prevalent for many reasons – but I think I had a lot of thoughts about feeling this way that made things more difficult than they had to be. And having this course to prime my days really helped with just that.

Student 15

Before discussing my self-reflections about MMP, I would like to begin by expressing how much of a positive experience MMP has on my self-identity and on my outlook on my future career as a physician. While the WELL Office provides helpful counselling and guides for our own personal struggles, participating in a group session has allowed me to uncover feelings of how I see myself and the world and how my peers do so as well. As a student who has previously done yoga to find inner peace and relaxation, and a student who has visited the WELL Office in the past, I have always strived to be self-aware and to find congruence (although never formally explained). In fact, at the beginning of the course, I thought the guided mediations would be similar to what I always experienced in past formal guided awareness sessions. However, discussing feelings and running through exercises that challenge how I interact with my peers made the guided meditation sessions more challenging. I felt that I was always experiencing a new sensation each time. Prior to this course, I always felt the same sensations over my body during meditation, and now I can feel pain, numbness, or nothing where before I could feel a wave of energy. Ultimately, I feel these newfound sensations are reflective of the new insights I have gained regarding myself and my feelings including how I handle life stressors. During my experience with MMP, I had the opportunity to practice the STOP approach and to reflect on how this technique may guide my approach to patients. I now feel better prepared to better care for patients and address daily life stressors by stopping and taking a breath. By determining if I am lacking congruence or if I am become aware of underlying stressors, I now feel more capable of addressing a problem in a new light. I feel this lesson can be applied to my medical profession and my personal life. Prior to this course, I always felt I was in the blaming stance: I blamed my mom for our noisy neighbors, and I blamed my peers for not holding tutorials that were in-depth enough often. Once I started using the STOP approach, not only do I feel I have a less explosive relationship with my mom but I also feel I can approach my peers with less anger and more cooperation. There is nothing more valuable than learning a skill that brings inner peace. While those are just a few of my wonderful experiences in MMP, I would like to end my reflections of my experience of MMP by discussing one of the biggest insights I have made regarding my future as a physician. The ability to tolerate your humanity, as said by Dr. X, has been one of a few sayings that have resonated in my soul. Prior to this course, I always had difficulty seeing myself as a physician because I never felt I could meet the standards of the "perfect" medical student. But it wasn't that I couldn't see myself as a physician, it was that I could not accept the fact that I am human being and that a physician is not made in one day. Overall, this MMP experience has taught me that I must have patience when it comes to who I want to be and where I want to go. On that note, I would like to thank my peers, Dr. X, and Dr. Y for showing me this. And finally, I would like to thank myself.

Student 16

The Mindful Medical Practice (MMP) course did not meet my expectations. Initially, I thought the class would focus on the trendy new item in medical education: the concept "wellness." As medical students we can hardly go a day without hearing this word. Whether it is about a "wellness room" or a "wellness week" or a "wellness class" or the "WELL Office," the notion of wellness and the lack thereof in medical school have been emphasized throughout our education as much as any other clinical concept. The administration's definition of wellness remains elusive to me. Is it being fit? Is it not being stressed out? I found the general approaches towards teaching wellness (if there can even be such a thing) superfluous. One cannot simply do a 10-minute relaxation in class to be "well." An hour for exercise scheduled on the week of our exam, while it is undoubtedly good, it does not really address the underlying issues pertaining to why there is a lack of wellness in medicine and does not go far enough in teaching us about resilience and coping in the face of our ever-mounting stressors and tasks. You hear the advice "take time to work on yourself," "exercise and eat healthy," or "make sure to spend enough time with your friends and family" over and over. While well intended, I could not help but to feel contempt, as I recognize that inevitably there will come a time when we simply might not have the time and energy required to do all of these and to do them well. If it were that easy, we wouldn't need a wellness discussion spanning, so far, 2 years of medical education. So, when I arrived to MMP, I was skeptic and expected the class to be something akin to a group meditation, combined with readings about mindfulness and how to cope with depression (exploring available resources should we come to feel "unwell"). Thankfully, this was far from the truth. In MMP, I finally felt like we were identifying and reflecting on the realities faced by medical students head on: "suffering," "burn out," "unrealistic expectations," and the "coping mechanisms" we employ when we come to face our mortality, all delve into why someone might become unwell in medicine. Speaking about these with our peers in a guided discussion with an elder/mentor physician was invaluable. Our mentor has made mistakes and *we* will also make mistakes. I am worried about clerkship and about my performance, just like the person sitting next to me. It served to humanize medicine and our role within it, and it helped normalize feelings towards the future. Most importantly, it helped me understand the effective and ineffective stances I might use to try to cope with future stressors and demands. The machinery that is medical school has a long legacy of being beautiful but ruthless, and it has no intention of meeting any of our expectations or for that matter, changing its wiring for our generation. While there has been movement towards changing the culture of medical education, ultimately our craft will demand we give up sleep, relationships, and attendance to social events. I knew this when I applied to medical school. There are arduous times ahead, but by providing us with tools to deal with the feelings that will inevitably arise, this 8-week class has done more for me than the wellness component of our curriculum has been able to do so far.

Student 17

I was really looking forwards to this course and was thankfully not disappointed. A couple of factors made this course amazing to me.

First of all, the fact that the course was scheduled on a Friday morning allowed me to utilize this course to the fullest by reflecting on my week during each class and starting the weekend on a positive note. That being said, not all the classes ended on a positive note to me. In fact, classes five and six (building resilience, being with suffering and mindful congruent practice in clerkship and beyond) were actually very difficult to go through without being challenged by some intense emotions.

Second of all, I loved our group! I thought that everyone was eager to participate which gave rise to great discussions. When FMD ended, I had a feeling that I knew everyone in the program, but I was most certainly wrong. During our first MMP class, I realized that I didn't know half the people in the class very well. By the end of the last class, I can ensure that I have at least five more good friends, thanks to this class.

Third of all, the content of the course itself was actually new to me, and I truly learnt a lot of theory which allowed me to learn more about myself. For instance, I learnt that I tend to placate a lot, where I disregard the self. But most importantly, I learnt that, to a patient, a doctor who is placating is not good just as a doctor who is blaming or computer-mind-ing. I thought, before attending MMP classes, that a doctor who validates a patient to the fullest and apologizes to the patient without giving too much of his opinion not to bother the patient is the best doctor. This class made me learn (through the exercise with different students acting out different stances) that a doctor should also give something of him/herself. Patients come to see the doctor for their expert opinion. As silly and obvious as this sound, it actually took me some time to understand this concept. A doctor who is merely mirroring the patient's wants without actually giving their opinion is not efficient and doesn't allow any progression in the treatment plan. This does not mean that I should blame myself or be mad at myself for placating if I ever do placate, but instead, this course has taught me to catch myself placating. By being aware of the stances I am taking in different situation, I am becoming more and more congruent (I believe). By taking a short break to realize that I am taking a placating stance and disregarding the self, I am taking the first step to becoming more mindful. Thus, the biggest lesson I have learnt is that being mindful allows me to take a second to think about what is going on in order to be as aware as possible of myself in order to make better decisions.

Fourth of all, I loved how each class started and ended with a short meditation session. As was mentioned by Dr. X, the more one practices meditation, the better one becomes at it. I have definitely seen an improvement in my meditations, in that I am distracted less often in the same span of time. Also, I have learnt to not beat myself up when I get distracted, instead to notice it as soon as possible and slowly bring back my attention to, for example, the toe we are asked to focus on.

Student 18

I'm not going to lie to you, Dr. X, I really did not expect this class to be so profoundly impactful. In fact, I was dreading attending the first class. I had been feeling quite disenchanted with medical school and aggravated by the intensity and passion that my peers seemed to exude, and I seemed to lack altogether. I was not interested in hearing their carefully crafted responses to your questions, and I was even less interested in sharing my own feelings, especially because most of them resembled inadequacy in one way or another. I had planned to stay quiet and keep to myself, as it seemed better not to share anything than to feign confidence and strength. I decided to participate for three reasons. Firstly, the setup of the class made it nearly impossible to disengage; the circle we sat in and the lack of a desk to hide my phone under meant I just as could see everyone at once, they too could see me. Secondly, you somehow found a way to make every single person in the room feel that you heard, understood, and valued their opinions. Thirdly, and most importantly by far, my peers proved me entirely wrong by sharing real feelings about real concerns. Their willingness to be vulnerable made me want to be vulnerable, too. I am so grateful that my mindset changed and that I was ultimately open enough to let the messages sink in and have an impact on my life.

In hindsight, I think I was struggling with depression at the start of the block. My aunt, who basically raised me until I was 8 years old, has become morbidly ill over the last few years and nearly died before Christmas. She is on a path to regaining her independence that will take years of hard work, both emotionally and physically, and I was overwhelmed with the burden of her disease. I am the daughter she never had and one of few people who truly understands her and loves her unconditionally, and I felt I could not take a step back to check in with my own feelings about the situation. I realize now that I was unable to distinguish between all the emotions I was feeling; fear, sadness, frustration, anger, despair, guilt, and intense longing for her recovery all manifested as me being unempathetic and callous with her. By participating in this class, I was able to confront all of these different emotions in contexts other than her illness and accept them as a part of my own process of coping and not just as negative and inappropriate. In learning not to judge myself for feeling the way I did, I was able to reframe the situation and change my outlook for the better. This class has given us real tools to deal not only with the demands of being a physician but also with the ups and downs of our personal relationships. It is an important part of our curriculum, and I want to thank you for investing time in our present and future well-being.

Appendix A. Mindful Movement Sequence (for use with Chap. 5, Class 3)

Mountain Pose
1. Stand with feet together or hip-width apart, parallel. Lift up the toes, spread them wide, and place them back on the floor. Feel your weight evenly balanced through the bottom of each foot, not leaning forwards or backwards.
2. Pull up the knee caps, squeeze the thighs, and tuck the tailbone slightly under. Feel the hips aligned directly over the ankles. The legs are straight, but the knees are not locked.
3. Inhale and lift out of the waist, pressing the crown of the head up towards the ceiling, feeling the spine long and straight.
4. Exhale and drop the shoulders down and back as you reach the fingertips towards the floor. Gently press the chest/sternum towards the front of the room.
5. Continue breathing and hold position for 4–8 breaths.

Shoulder Rotations
1. Stand with feet shoulder-width apart.
2. Inhale and bring shoulders up to the ears.
3. Exhale and roll shoulders back and down.
4. Repeat 3–4 times.
5. Repeat steps 2–4 in the opposite direction.

Lateral Neck Stretches (or Neck Rolls)
1. Stand with feet hip-width apart, arms by the sides.
2. Hold your left wrist with your right hand behind your back.
3. Inhale and use right hand to gently straighten your left arm and pull down slightly.
4. Exhale and slowly lower your right ear towards your right shoulder only as far as is comfortable, feeling the stretch in the left side of your neck.
5. Hold for 30 seconds. Keep breathing.
6. Switch sides and repeat steps 2–5.

Side Bends
1. Stand with feet hip-width apart.
2. Inhale and bring your right arm up and stretch towards the ceiling.
3. Exhale and bend gently to the left. Keep your chin parallel to floor and feel the stretch in your side.
4. Inhale back to center.
5. Repeat steps 2–4 lifting your left arm up and bending to the right.

© Springer Nature Switzerland AG 2020
S. Liben, T. A. Hutchinson, *MD Aware*,
https://doi.org/10.1007/978-3-030-22430-1

Rag Doll Forward Bend
   1. Stand with feet hip-width apart, arms relaxed at sides.
   2. Inhale and bring your arms up over your head.
   3. Exhaling release down and bend slowly forwards at the hips. Allow your knees to bend slightly as you move into a relaxed forward bend.
   4. Allow your arms/hands and head to relax completely, hanging loose like a rag doll. Arms can dangle or can clasp together at the elbows if more comfortable.
   5. May gently sway front to back or side to side. Hold position for several breaths.
   6. Inhale and SLOWLY come back up to standing, one vertebra at a time.

Mountain Pose (See Instructions Above)

Appendix B. Role play cards (for use with Chap. 6, Class 4)

Front	Back

Placating Stance	*Placating Stance*
	     Doing everything you can to please the patient
	     Give up your own values and your own agenda
	     Tell the patient what he/she wants to hear
	 Your job is to interview this patient using this stance

Blaming Stance	*Blaming Stance*
	     Make it clear the patient needs to meet your expectations
	     Use the word "should" a lot
	     Some anger and impatience directed at the patient
	 Your job is to interview this patient using this stance

S. Liben, T. A. Hutchinson, *MD Aware*,
https://doi.org/10.1007/978-3-030-22430-1

Front	Back

Super-Reasonable Stance
 	
Self   Other   Context
	Super-Reasonable Stance
	   In your head. Not feeling or acknowledging your own or patient's emotions
	   Dealing purely with facts and data
	   Focus on analysis and thinking
	Your job is to interview this patient using this stance

Distracting Stance
 	
Self   Other   Context
	Distracting Stance
	   Your mind is off somewhere else – hard time focusing on this patient
	   Multitasking during the interview
	   Inappropriate humor
	Your job is to interview this patient using this stance

Congruence
 	
Self   Other   Context
	Congruence
	   Respectfully present to yourself and to the other person
	   Engaged and listening but also expressing your own perspective
	   Empathetic but/and attempting to move things forwards
	Your job is to interview this patient while being congruent

KAREN	A diabetic woman who is now in her 50s, she was a model when in her 20s and now has a severely ischemic right leg. This has been treated in a variety of ways with no success and she now needs a below-knee amputation. She does not want the amputation although it is the medically indicated course of action Your job is to play this patient

Appendix C. Iceberg metaphor (for use with Chap. 9, Class 7)

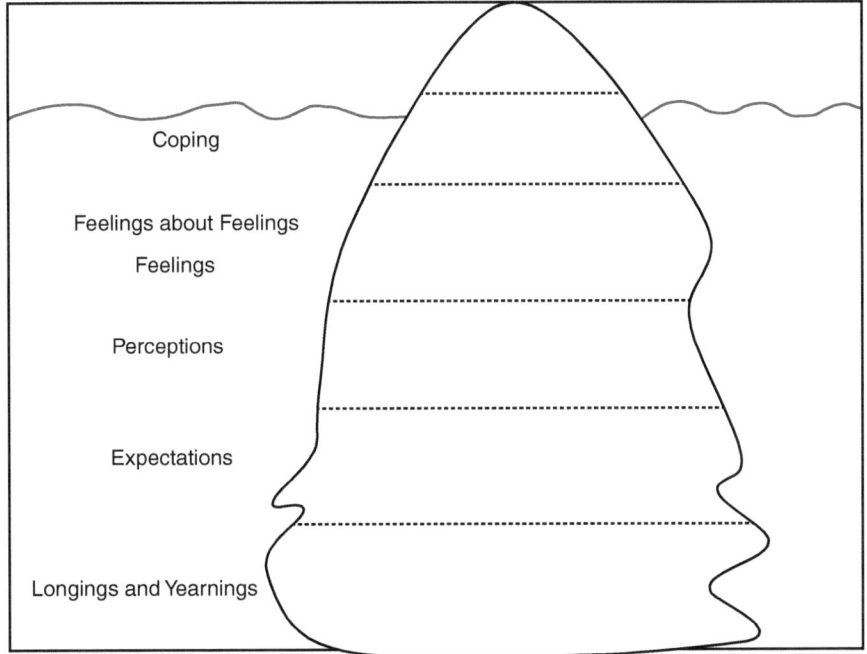

Coping

Feelings about Feelings

Feelings

Perceptions

Expectations

Longings and Yearnings

Appendix D. "Fire" by Judy Brown (for use with Chap. 9, Class 7)

What makes a fire burn
is space between the logs,
a breathing space.
Too much of a good thing,
too many logs
packed in too tight
can douse the flames
almost as surely
as a pail of water would.
So building fires
requires attention
to the spaces in between,
as much as to the wood.
When we are able to build
open spaces
in the same way
we have learned
to pile on the logs,
then we can come to see how
it is fuel, and absence of the fuel
together, that make fire possible.
We only need to lay a log
lightly from time to time.
A fire
grows
simply because the space is there,
with openings
in which the flame
that knows just how it wants to burn
can find its way.

Reprinted from: Brown J. A leader's guide to reflective practice. Bloomington: Trafford Publishing; 2006.

Appendix E. Tips for Mindful Practices (for use with Chap. 9, Class 7)

Formal Practices

1. Take 10 minutes (set a timer) each weekday morning or evening at a set time to practice a seated guided awareness exercise. Guided awareness practices are available on the internet. It may be helpful to set up a small space in your house or apartment for this daily practice.
2. Make a plan to eat one meal per week slowly, and in silence, with no Internet or other stimulation. Use your awareness to experience each bite.
3. Use a mindful walking practice when you are waiting in slow-moving lines.
4. Consider going on a 5–7 day meditation retreat.

Informal Practices

1. Use S.T.O.P. (stop, take a breath, observe, proceed) when you are feeling rushed or stressed.
2. Each time you settle into a chair, take a moment to bring awareness to your feet, then legs, then hands, and up to the top of your head.
3. Use "waiting times" (e.g., in long lines, at the airport) to bring awareness to your body sensations.
4. If you notice that you are in one of the unhelpful Satir stances, such as placating, blaming, or being super-reasonable, see if you can make room to include aspects of the experience you might be leaving out.
5. In the moments when you notice that you have failed to be mindful and find yourself acting out reactively, remember that you are now being mindful and be gentle in your own self-judgment.
6. It is neither easy nor necessary to do everything on your own – seek out help and guidance from others whom you trust.

© Springer Nature Switzerland AG 2020
S. Liben, T. A. Hutchinson, *MD Aware*,
https://doi.org/10.1007/978-3-030-22430-1

Appendix F. Notes for Students

MMP Class 1: Attention and Awareness

What is the MMP course and how does it apply to the practice of medicine?
The MMP course is a small group participatory experiential learning course given over seven consecutive weeks. The course integrates contemplative practices (e.g., guided attention) with specific topics for the seven classes that each apply to a specific area of clinical practice such as medical errors, challenging communication skills, resilience, and how to facilitate helpful responses to suffering.

Why is MMP being offered just prior to clerkship?
Just before being immersed in the world of clinical medicine via clerkship is an opportune time for the acquisition and honing of specific clinical skills.

What two broad skills is the MMP course looking to impart to students?
1. To learn and practice specific clinical skills to help students better *care for their patients*
2. To have students learn and practice how to build resilience and *better care for themselves* as they care for others

Change Blindness

A surprising perceptual phenomenon that occurs when a change in a visual stimulus is introduced that the observer does not notice despite being forewarned that a change will take place. For example, observers often fail to notice a major change in a static image as one part of the image dissolves into another. Such "change blindness" may reflect fundamental limitations of human attention. Limits and lapses in attention (visual attention being one small part of overall attentional capacity) may underlie many medical errors (e.g., lack of situational awareness).

© Springer Nature Switzerland AG 2020
S. Liben, T. A. Hutchinson, *MD Aware*,
https://doi.org/10.1007/978-3-030-22430-1

Guided Awareness Practices (Meditation)

Mindfulness (mindful awareness) can be cultivated by guided (or unguided) awareness practices while sitting, standing, lying down, or walking.

Awareness of Red Exercise

Forcing a decision between two choices (e.g., red or not red) brings out the arbitrariness involved in categorizing objects and experiences as this or that. While making binary choices is important in medical practice (e.g., deciding whether a lumbar puncture is required or not), so is the awareness of the influences and biases that undergird such decisions.

"Something Missed" Narrative Exercise

Paying full conscious attention, at all times, to what is being said and not said in any interaction is beyond the limits of human attentional capacity. Recognizing the limits of attention can serve as motivation to learn ways to improve attentional capacity, such as practicing guided awareness.

Cellphone Exercise

The idea of "multitasking" may be a myth as there is increasing evidence that rather than being able to multitask many things at the same time in parallel, attention instead jumps from one point of focus to another in series. Even if multitasking proves to be possible, the experience of being only partially listened to is less than satisfying. Physicians can always choose to bring their full attention to their patients as one way to foster good doctor-patient relationships. Additionally, as will be experienced in Class 5 (Chap. 7), paying full attention to patients is also more satisfying and meaningful for the physician themselves.

MMP Class 2: Congruent Communication

Reacting Versus Responding

- *Reaction (R)*: An automatic and unchosen way of relating to another person or stimulus
- *Response (RS)*: A conscious and chosen way of relating to another person or stimulus

1. Reacting: Unconscious reaction to a stimulus (S) – one stimulus results in one possible reaction (R)

$$S \rightarrow R$$

Versus

2. Responding: Conscious response to a stimulus – one stimulus, with a mindful pause, results in several possible responses (RS)

$$
\begin{aligned}
S \; + \; \textbf{MINDFUL PAUSE} \;\; &\rightarrow \;\; \textbf{RS} \\
&\rightarrow \;\; \textbf{RS} \\
&\rightarrow \;\; \textbf{RS} \\
&\rightarrow \;\; \textbf{RS}
\end{aligned}
$$

What creates the possibilities of many RS versus only one R?
A Mindful Pause. The awareness to pause and reassess when it feels like there might be only way to react, using this mindful pause to see other options of how to respond instead, and then making a conscious mindful choice of what to do out of all the options available.

Communication Stances

Family therapist Virginia Satir identified three elements in any interaction between two people (self, other, and context).

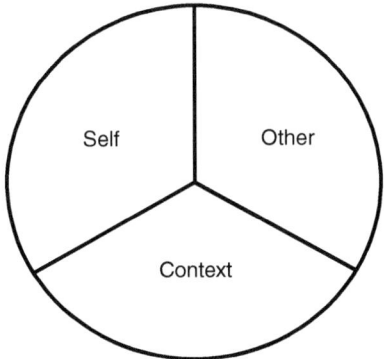

Elements of an interaction between two people

Satir also identified four common unconscious stances that people tend to adopt that leave out elements in the interaction. The part left out is indicated by shading in the diagrams below.

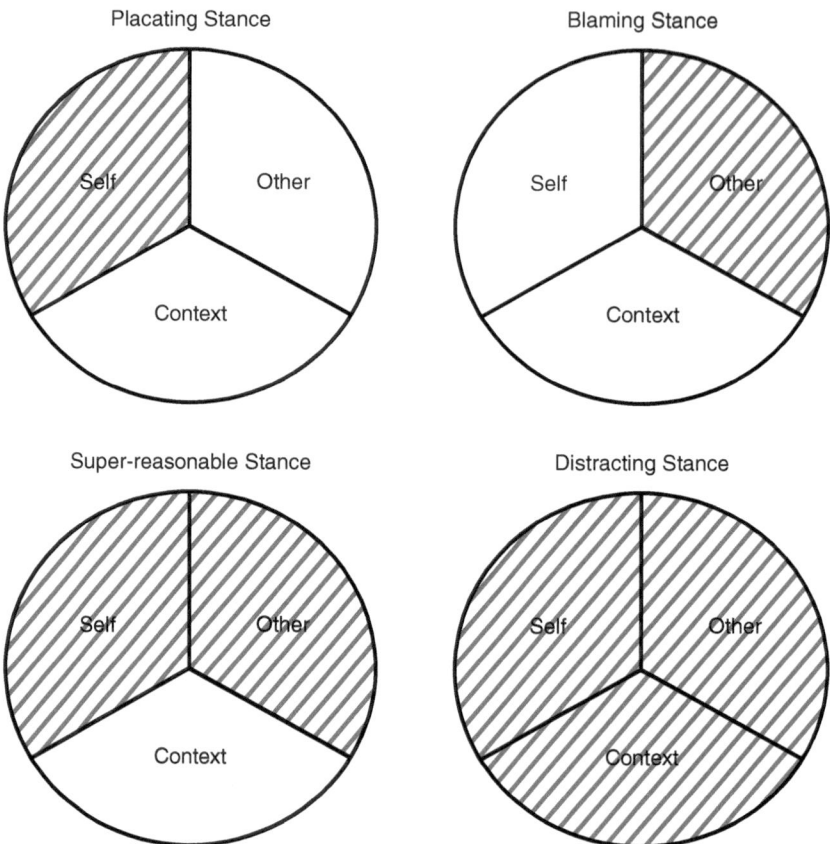

Finally, there is a physical posture associated with each stance, which are also shown below: placating on one knee, right hand over heart, left hand reaching up; blaming with left hand on hip and right hand pointing at the other person; the super-reasonable looking above the other person in a superior way; distracting has many ways to be portrayed and we did not act it out in class.

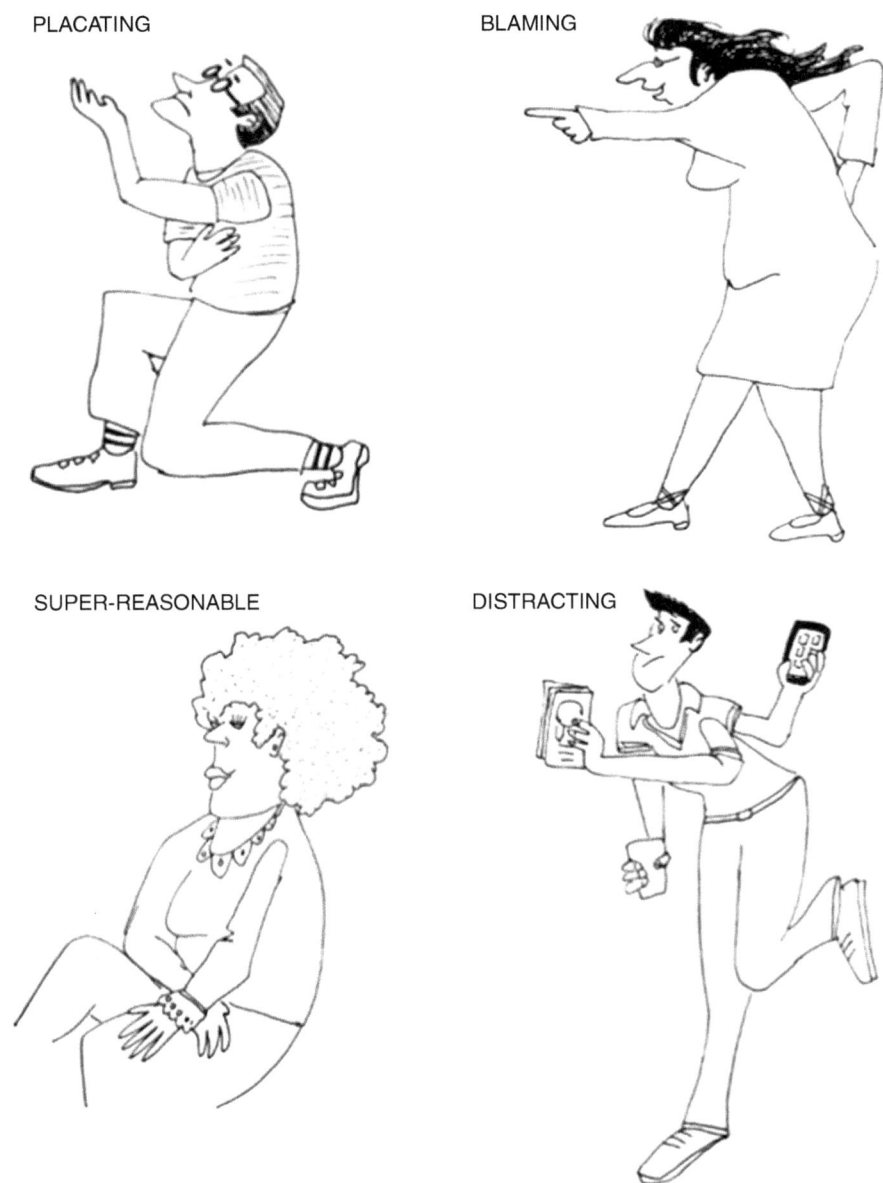

PLACATING

BLAMING

SUPER-REASONABLE

DISTRACTING

Adapted by Chris Tucker from Satir V. The new peoplemaking. Mountain View: Science and Behavior Books; 1988.

The ideal way that Satir recommended in relating to another person is congruence, where all of the elements are included.

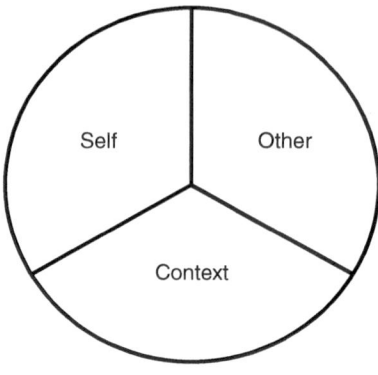

Congruence

The relationship of mindfulness to these stances is that mindfulness allows us to create a pause, notice what is being left out, and then make a choice about how to proceed. This might mean putting back in the missing awareness (of self, other, or context) in order to produce congruence, or it might mean a choice to continue in a stance. In either case, we have turned an automatic reaction into a chosen response.

MMP Class 3: Awareness and Decision-Making

Formal Awareness Practice (Meditation)

Formal cultivation of mindful awareness is when the practice of attention focuses on a bodily sensation at set times and for defined durations within protected spaces. These formal practices may be done while sitting, standing, walking, or lying down and most often focus attention on a body sensation such as the breath.

Informal Awareness Practice

Informal practice is when attention is briefly placed on a body sensation (such as the breath) at unplanned times of the day, for brief undefined durations, and within everyday activities such as while washing hands or walking from one place to another.

Iowa Gambling Experiment (Four Decks of Cards)

This study used galvanic skin responses (hand sweating) to examine the correlation between somatic unconscious changes and conscious awareness of decision-making while choosing a winning or losing card. Subjects were found to have increased hand sweating (indicating a stress response) much earlier than when they became consciously aware of making a losing card (bad) choice. The study highlights the conscious and unconscious processes that occur in decision-making and that we are not fully consciously aware of when we make decisions.

Medical Errors Video: "Just a Routine Operation": https://www.youtube. com/watch?v=JzlvgtPIof4

Some of the kinds of errors seen in the video include:

- Lack of situational awareness
- Lack of clarity of lines of communication
- Lack of closed loop communication
- Lack of assertiveness
- Unclear who was in charge of effecting decisions

While we do not know what the galvanic stress response was for the clinicians involved in the medical error scenario, it is likely that many were aware, on some conscious level, that the situation was out of control. Preventing medical errors not only requires moment-to-moment self-awareness of thoughts, emotions, and body sensations but also the awareness of self, other, and context in order to affect changes through effective behavioral stances (e.g., congruent Satir stance).

Mindful Movement

Intentionally bringing attention to body sensations during guided movements (e.g., yoga) is another way to practice focusing attention and increasing mindful awareness. Increased capacity to pay attention to internal sensations may serve as additional sources of information during stressful potentially error-causing situations.

MMP Class 4: Clinical Congruence

Below is a diagram of physician, patient, and disease.

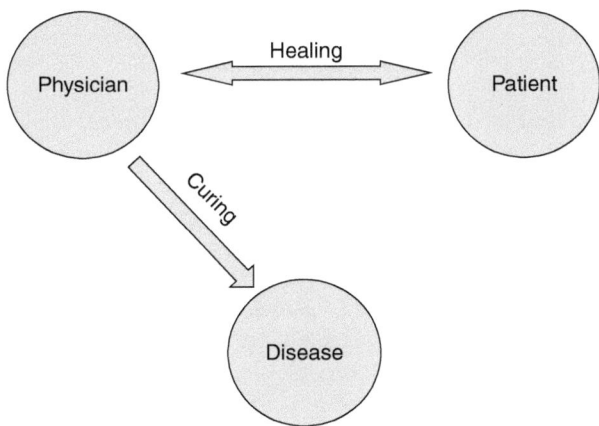

The separation of the disease from the patient by the process of diagnosis is important for patients: relief of responsibility and empowerment. It is also important for physicians: pragmatic (it is how we organize information and our thinking about the biology of the disease); we need to do two simultaneous and different jobs at the same time – to fix or cure and to promote healing.

When we superimpose the self, other, and context diagram on the physician, patient, and disease diagram, we get the results shown below.

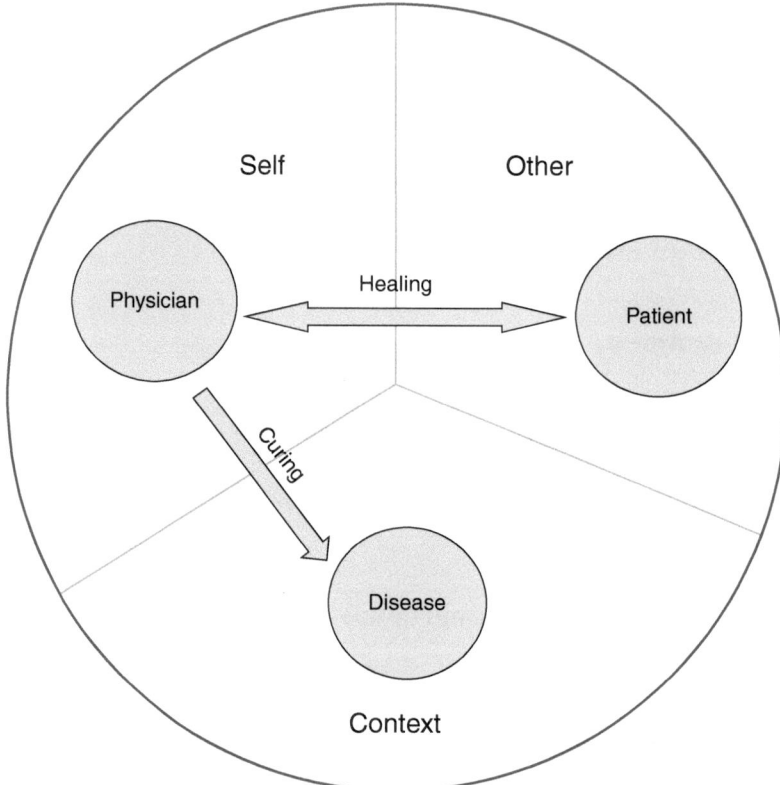

When we act out the communication stances in a clinical context, as we did in class, we tend to act and communicate in the ways described below for each stance.

Placating Stance

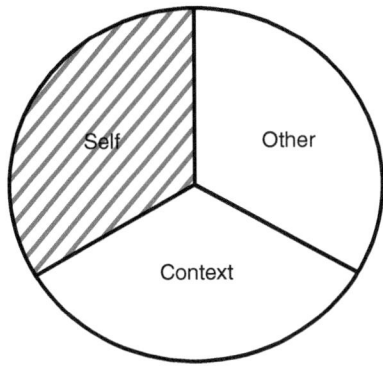

- Doing everything you can to please the patient
- Give up your own values and your own agenda
- Tell the patient what they want to hear

Blaming Stance

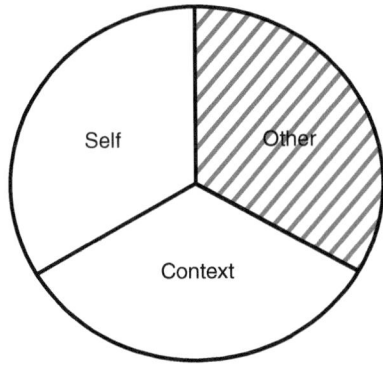

- Make it clear the patient needs to meet your expectations
- Use the word "should" a lot
- Some anger and impatience directed at the patient

Super-Reasonable Stance

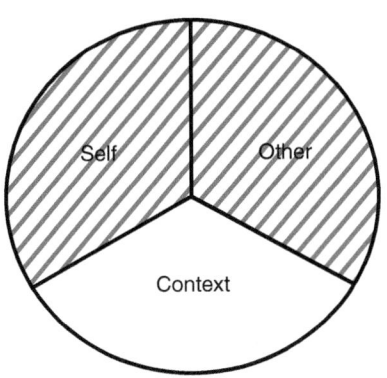

- In your head. Not feeling or acknowledging your own or patient's emotions
- Dealing purely with facts and data
- Focus on analysis and thinking

Distracting Stance

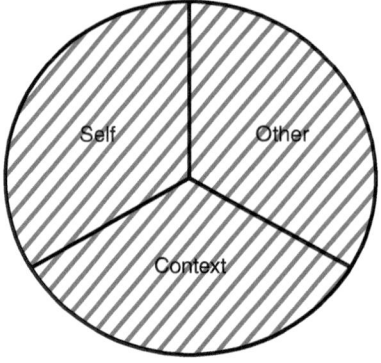

- Your mind is off somewhere else – hard time focusing on this patient
- Multitasking during the interview
- Inappropriate humor

Congruence

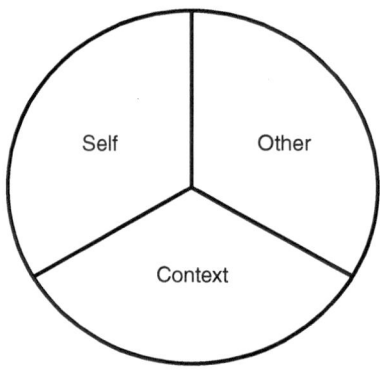

- Respectfully present to yourself and to the other person
- Engaged and listening but also expressing your own perspective
- Empathetic but/and attempting to move things forwards

The Three As

The three As stand for awareness, acceptance or allowing, and action. The reason to stress these three is that usually or frequently we move immediately from awareness to action without taking time to accept or allow what has happened. Part of the purpose of teaching mindfulness is to allow us to rest for a moment in the accepting or allowing mode. This gives us a moment to choose how to proceed but also allows us to act more powerfully. Contrary to our initial impression, acceptance does not lead to resignation but to a more grounded and more effective response to whatever we are facing.

MMP Class 5: Building Resilience

Listening Awareness Exercise

Bringing attention to sounds in the room (or to music being played) is another way to practice paying attention in the cultivation of mindful awareness. Bringing awareness to whether we "like, do not like, or are indifferent" to particular sounds may be helpful as practice to be aware of biases of "liking or not liking" certain kinds of patient stories. By bringing awareness to our "liking or not liking" specific patients, we can be more open to being curious as to the reasons for these preferences and in turn be less judgmental and more open.

Triangle of Attention

As we have seen for ourselves in guided awareness practices, we can bring attention to any of the three aspects of subjective experience: (1) thoughts, (2) physical sensations, or (3) emotions. Because physical sensations are always grounded in the present moment (e.g., we feel a toothache only when it is present and cannot re-experience the painful sensation once it is over), bringing attention to the breath from moment to moment can serve as an ever-present "anchor" to bring our attention back to what is actually happening right now, rather than to thoughts or emotions over what will happen in the future or what happened in the past.

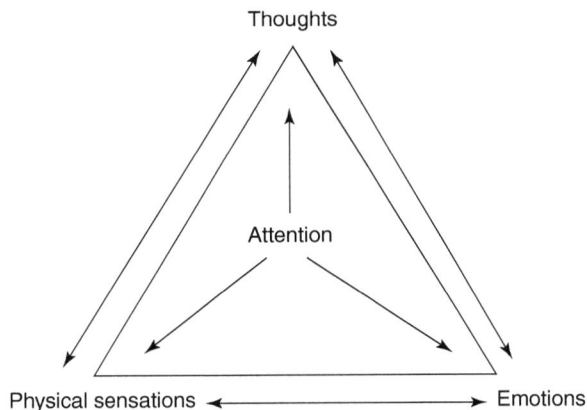

Definition of Mindfulness

The awareness that emerges by paying attention, moment to moment, in a particular way (nonjudgmentally). This awareness may be cultivated by specific guided and unguided formal and informal awareness practices.

Definition of Burnout (Mostly affects work rather than home life)

1. Emotional exhaustion
2. Depersonalization
3. Lack sense of accomplishment

Psychological Resilience

- An individual's ability to adapt to stress and adversity.
- Is a process rather than a fixed trait.
- Can be developed and improved upon like other learnable skills.
- Resilience does not mean the absence of negative thoughts & emotions, but rather the capacity to allow whatever arises to be as it is, to not be resisted or suppressed.

Resilience Zone (The Area Between the Two Horizontal Lines in the Figures Below)

- The resilience zone is not fixed and varies within a person over time. Our capacity to be within the resilience zone depends on a multiplicity of factors some of which are under conscious control (e.g., pausing to eat when hungry can increase resilience).
- Mindful awareness allows for recognition of when we are at the upper or lower limits of our resilience zone. Once aware we can then pause to determine what we can do to bring ourselves back into the zone.

The Resilient Zone

In the "Resilient Zone" individuals have the best capacity for:
Flexibility and adaptability
Pro-social behavior
Executive functioning
Being responsive rather than reactive

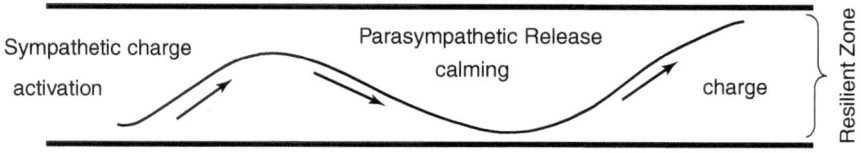

Individuals can learn to remain in and return to the Resilient Zone

S.T.O.P Exercise: An Informal Awareness Practice

1. *S*top.
2. *T*ake (or be aware of) a breath.

3. *O*bserve (what is going on externally, i.e., the context, as well as the internal thoughts, emotions, and physical sensations).
4. *P*roceed (that may mean taking a specific action or not taking any action).

Deep Listening Exercise (As Practiced in Dyads)

By mindfully grounding thoughts, emotions, and physical sensations in the present moment, and by not interrupting when someone is talking, it is possible to listen deeply to another person. Deep listening is valued by both the listener and the speaker (equivalent to the clinician and the patient). For the speaker, being heard is felt as an act of compassion and caring and is helpful in and of itself. For the listener, bringing full attention to the speaker allows space for trust and caring to emerge in relationship. This type of listening promotes connection, is beneficial to both involved, and is an antidote to the burnout triad of emotional exhaustion, depersonalization, and lack sense of accomplishment.

Deep listening is proactive and can always be done with and for patients, no matter what the diagnosis or prognosis. The clinician who understands the power of deep listening would never feel the need to think or say to a patient that there is "nothing more that can be done."

MMP Class 6: Responding to Suffering

Pain and Suffering

Pain is the initial automatic (or reflexive) unpleasant physical sensation or emotional reaction that arises either when we get what is not wanted (e.g., physical pain) or don't get what we want (e.g., money or status). Physical pain sensations do not necessarily always result in the experience of suffering (e.g., pain felt during exercise).

Suffering results from how we interpret or relate to actual or perceived threats to the integrity of any of the domains of experience that include the physical, emotional, social, economic, existential, and religious. Pain arises as a reflex and is an inevitable part of life, while suffering is how we relate to the pain we are experiencing. Suffering results from the stories we tell ourselves about our pain. Another way to express the difference between pain and suffering is to say that suffering results from our resistance to pain.

Responses to suffering can be unhelpful (e.g., blaming, placating avoidance/abandonment, over-intellectualization) or helpful (e.g., deep listening, being present and congruent). Whether a response is helpful or unhelpful (or somewhere in between) will depend on the specific people involved and the context. Mindful awareness and being congruent helps discern how to best respond to suffering.

Awareness of Time Exercise

This exercise, which involves listing goals and dreams and revising the list based on an imagined shortened life expectancy (from 6 months to 1 day), is one way of highlighting how our priorities may change when we have an increased awareness of our own mortality. How we re-evaluate our priorities in life when there is less time to live has implications both for how we live our own lives, as well as how we perceive and respond to what is important to patients.

Mortality Salience

Mortality salience (MS) is a state in which an individual is reminded (consciously or unconsciously) that his or her death is inevitable. Increased mortality salience results in existential anxiety, which may be buffered by one's own cultural worldview and/or sense of self-esteem.

Terror Management Theory

Terror management theory (TMT) is based on the work of Ernest Becker and proposes a basic psychological conflict that results from having a desire to live but realizing that death is inevitable. This conflict produces existential terror and is believed to be unique to human beings. Moreover, the solution to the conflict is also generally unique to humans: culture and self-esteem.

According to TMT, cultures are symbolic systems that act to provide life with shared meaning and value, including shared worldviews, which offer literal (e.g., belief in an afterlife) and/or symbolic immortality (e.g., contributing to something greater or longer lasting than an individual's life).

Self-esteem, which TMT theorists define as the degree to which people believe they are meeting or exceeding cultural standards, is bolstered, and death anxiety is diminished when people believe that they are active and valued members of their respective cultures (and this can include the "medical culture" to which physicians belong).

Increased mortality salience has been shown to strengthen one's cultural worldviews and attempts to live up to culturally prescribed standards. This can affect a wide range of behaviors, including strengthening one's adherence to particular cultural norms (upholding cultural stereotypes and beliefs) as well as distancing from those who are different in their culture or worldview.

Healthcare professionals work in an environment of increased mortality salience. If not consciously aware of the biases thus evoked towards their own cultural group and away from the perceived "other," they may respond with unexamined adherence to the biomedical model and/or unhelpful distancing of the patient/other. On the other hand, if increased mortality salience is brought to conscious awareness, then more helpful responses to suffering become possible.

"Just Like Me" Exercise

Contemplation of the common human desires for health, safety, and happiness is one way to bring compassion to the care of everyone, not just to those we relate positively towards.

MMP Class 7: Mindful Congruent Practice in Clerkship and Beyond

Iceberg Metaphor

Yearnings and Longings Our most deeply held hopes, wishes, and desires such as to make a real difference, to be loved, and so on.

Expectations What you expect will happen or should happen.

Perceptions The meaning that you give to your longings, yearnings, expectations, and whatever else you are aware of. This might include "This is a worthwhile activity," "I wish I was doing something else," "This has been a good experience," etc.

Feelings Feelings such as anxiety, joy, anger/resentment, fear, gratitude, and so on.

Feelings About Feelings We don't just have feelings; we have feelings about those feelings. We may be anxious about our feelings, grateful for them, fear them, and so on.

Coping/Stances We adopt our stances primarily in relation to our own feelings about our feelings. We may suppress those feelings (placating); project them (blaming); completely deny them (super reasonable); check out as completely as we can (irrelevant/distracting); or acknowledge, accept, and be present to them (congruent).

Four Levels of Knowing (e.g. knowledge of personal mortality)

1. *Not knowing*: "?"
2. *Knowing*: "While I know that I will die (someday), I don't live my day-to-day life any differently…"
3. *Realizing*: "Oh, so this universal truth that death is for everyone, including me, truly applies to me also…!?"
4. *Actualizing*: "Deeply knowing that i too will die I live my life differently moment to moment…"

Index

© Springer Nature Switzerland AG 2020
S. Liben, T. A. Hutchinson, *MD Aware*,
https://doi.org/10.1007/978-3-030-22430-1